Praise for MENtal Health

Every story shared chips away at the silence men have carried for generations. When we see our own struggles in another man's experience, we realize we're not alone — and this book lights the way.

— *Michael Pund, Founder of Wingman Mental Health*

Any man will see some aspect of himself in these stories of struggle, shame, vulnerability, and healing. This book is an invitation to step beyond the old definitions of masculinity shaped by families, cultures, and societies, and discover a more authentic, connected, and hopeful way of living. It's not only for men, but for anyone who cares about them—and the relationships that grow richer when men are free to embrace their true selves.

— *David Letiecq, MA, LPC, LCPC Letiecq Coaching, Counseling & Consulting www.letiecq.com*

The courage, heart and hope contained in these writings bring light to the dark places where men often get lost. If you are a man, if you love a man, if you have a father, brother or son, please read this book.

These are the perspectives of several men and women that have been through the fires, emerged better for (or despite) it, and are now open to sharing. I encourage you to read their stories for a healthier relationship with the men in your life.

— *Paul L. Symmonds, LCSW (Retired)*

Raw and honest vignettes that challenge outdated socially constructed norms of masculinity through avenues of vulnerability, self-reflection and authentic connections with others.

— *Dr. Will Folberth, PsyD*

MENtal Health is a series of revelatory stories of men grappling with mental illness, sexuality, abuse, violence, shame and most of all - lack of emotional support - and finding their True Selves in the process. Hopefully this brave collection will give other men permission to face and share their own struggles.

Highly recommended for all men and the women who love them.

— *Mimi Rich, Ma. Licensed Marriage and Family Therapist & Award-winning Author of* Feisty

MENtal Health is a powerful collection of stories from men across the globe finding themselves and creating better connections in the world as a human. The men in these stories are men you know - your father, brother, co-worker, partner - and they are all craving for the human connection while battling the traditional 'masculine' roles handed down through the generations and social programming. These men are lovingly sharing their light through the dark patriarchal maze so we can all better human together.

— *Brandee Melcher, Award Winning Author of* The Break: Rediscovering Our Inner Knowing.

MENtal Health: Take It "Like a Man," brings together a wide range of voices, social workers, therapists, coaches, veterans, writers, and everyday men who share deeply personal accounts of their struggles with masculinity, silence, trauma, and healing. The book is less about solutions and more about testimony. Each chapter feels like a window into a different man's life, revealing how cultural expectations, family systems, addiction, sexuality, grief, and love shape the ways men understand themselves. The foreword frames the project as a bold act of truth-telling, and the stories that follow hold nothing back. They are raw, painful, and at times surprisingly tender.

What struck me most while reading was the honesty. These stories feel unfiltered, which made me lean in closer. I found myself pausing often because the emotions resonated with me. The book reminded me of late-night conversations that don't come easy but stick with you long after. Some chapters were almost too heavy to read, yet that heaviness was part of the point. It made me think about how much men keep hidden and how damaging that silence can be.

Contributors offered beautifully crafted narratives that flowed like memoirs. Men's mental health isn't neat or orderly. It's complicated, jagged, and layered. The diversity of voices actually reinforces that truth. Chapter 6, "You Are Not Alone," was one of my favorites because of the way it spoke directly to the reader with warmth and reassurance. I liked how the chapter cut through the stigma and reminded men that isolation is not the answer, even when shame or fear makes it feel that way.

By the time I finished, I felt moved and hopeful. *MENtal Health* is not an easy book, and it isn't meant to be. I would recommend it to anyone who wants to understand the invisible burdens men carry. It's especially powerful for those who work with men in counseling, education, or leadership, as well as partners, siblings, or friends who want to listen better. What you'll find is an open invitation to break the silence and begin healing.

— *Literary Titan*

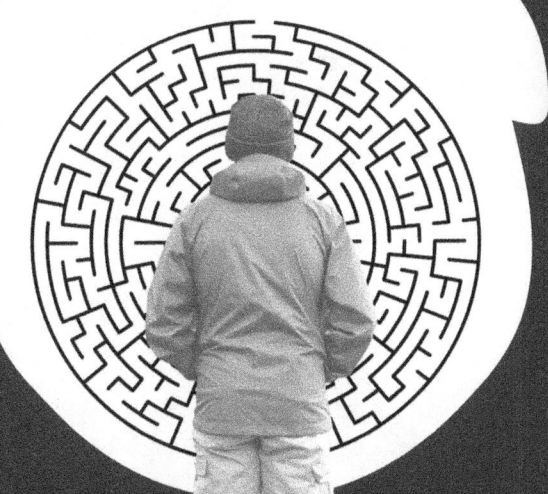

MENtal Health

Take It "Like a Man"

Eric Campos   Jason Schneider   Joshua Engle
Coach Zeke   Juan Camilo Posada Arenas
Christen E. Bryce   Federico Soto   Alan James Duro
Roje Khalique   Dr. Stacey Kevin Frick
Steven A. Schechter   Marc Longwith
Dr. Vincent Johnson Jr.   Jonathan Dubrulle
Natalie Goodfellow   Sierra Melcher

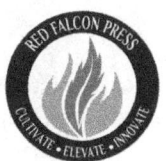

Copyright © 2025 by Red Falcon Press

All rights reserved.

No part of this book may be reproduced in any form or by any electronic or mechanical means, including information storage and retrieval systems, without written permission from the author, except for the use of brief quotations in a book review.

Red Thread Publishing LLC. 2025

Write to **info@redthreadbooks.com** if you are interested in publishing with Red Thread Publishing. Learn more about publications or foreign rights acquisitions of our catalog of books: www.redthreadbooks.com

ISBN Paperback: 979-8-89294-037-5

ISBN Hardcover: 979-8-89294-041-2

ISBN Ebook: 979-8-89294-038-2

DISCLAIMER:

The information and advice contained in this book are based upon the research and the personal and professional experiences of the authors. Some names and characteristics have been changed, some events have been compressed, and some dialogue has been recreated. Chapters reflect the authors' present recollections of experiences over time. The opinions herein are of each individual contributor. All writings are the property of individual contributors.

The publisher and authors are not responsible for any adverse effects or consequences resulting from the use of any of the suggestions, preparations, or procedures discussed in this book.

Contents

Foreword Sierra Melcher	xi
1. THE MAN THEY MADE, THE BOY THEY BROKE Eric Campos	1
2. A DIFFERENT KIND OF HARD Jason Schneider	12
3. I THOUGHT I WAS TOO SUCCESSFUL TO BE AN ADDICT Joshua Engle	22
4. THE HIDDEN DETERMINANTS Coach Zeke	33
5. WHAT, MENTAL HEALTH? Juan Camilo Posada Arenas	50
6. YOU ARE NOT ALONE Christen E. Bryce, RN, MS	57
7. HOW TO BE A CREATIVE WHILE STAYING (SORTA) SANE Federico Soto	64
8. MISSION ACCEPTED Alan James Duro	77
9. BREAKING THE CODE Roje Khalique	85
10. A PARADIGM SHIFT IN MEN'S MENTAL HEALTH Dr. Stacey Kevin Frick	102
11. SUCH A HEAVY LOAD Steven A. Schechter	111
12. DICHOTOMY Marc Longwith	122
13. MENIFEST Dr. Vincent Johnson Jr.	140
14. BEAUTY OUT OF ASHES Jonathan Dubrulle	158
15. FOR THE LOVE OF MEN Natalie Goodfellow	170

Acknowledgements	181
Review this Book	183
Red Falcon Press	185
Other books	187

Foreword
Sierra Melcher

Why is a Woman Writing the Foreword to a Book About Men's Mental Health? I've asked myself this question more than once over the nearly two years of bringing this project to life.

There are a few answers I could give:
   I'm the publisher and the one who initiated the project.
   It was my idea.
   I'm an award-winning author.

All of those points are true.
   But none of them are the reasons I said yes.
   I said yes because this book matters.
   Because men's mental health is not just a man's issue, it's a human one.
   Because I love men: my father, my partner, my friends, my brothers, my cousins, my son, and I have seen how often they suffer in silence.

This anthology is a courageous act. It is a container of truth. It is a space where men have gathered to speak the unspeakable, to say the things they were told to bury, to offer their stories not as finished tales but as starting points for healing.

Every book we publish is for the reader.
This one especially.
We came together with the shared purpose of making something often taboo, *men's mental health*, more visible, more spoken, and more real.
Because we can't heal what we're not allowed to name.
And we can't support what we refuse to see.

I don't claim to be an expert in men's mental health. The men who share their stories here are the true guides. They live this. They know what it costs to stay silent, and what it takes to speak up. And yet, you'll find women among the contributors, too. When we asked the men if this was appropriate, they said:

"Women are the mirrors in which we see ourselves."

"Our vulnerability is truly vulnerable when we are witnessed, especially by women."

Their insights floored me. And they reminded me that healing is relational.

We are all shaped in connection, and harmed there, too. Which means we all have a role to play in creating space for healing.

The *systemic and cultural weight* men carry to be strong, silent, and stoic isn't just theirs to bear; it's woven into the fabric of our culture. When we begin to unweave those threads, we free not only men, but everyone who loves them.

So this is my invitation, especially to women:
Let us listen without trying to fix.
Let us witness without needing men to be anything other than what they are.
Let us reflect on how our own words, expectations, or silences may have contributed to the pain of the men we love, not to blame ourselves, but to become more conscious participants in healing.

And to the men reading, ask yourselves:

How have I been part of the silence around men's mental health?
What would it mean to show up, fully, for myself?
What would it mean to let others see me as I am?

I don't come with answers. This book isn't about answers. It's about *truth*. And that, I've learned, is where healing begins. Throughout this journey, I've often referred to this project as *cool dudes talking about hard stuff*. But truly, it's so much more than that.

The men you will meet within these pages are not just co-authors or collaborators. I've come to know these individuals as the wise, courageous, and wildly generous humans they are. It was a privilege to watch them create something truly special by showing up to this project, not just for themselves and one another, but for you, dear reader. This book is a beginning.

May it be a spark.
May it be a mirror.
May it be a soft place to land.
Welcome.

— Sierra Melcher, CEO of Red Thread Publishing &
Red Falcon Press

Chapter 1

The Man They Made, the Boy They Broke

Eric Campos

I can still hear their voices—my biological father and uncles—each instructing me how to stand, laugh, walk, and even breathe. *Hold yourself like this. Speak deeper. Don't cry. Act like a man*, they'd say.

From my earliest memories, I wasn't just taught; I was molded and shaped into their vision of masculinity. Their gaze followed me everywhere—how I walked, stood, even how I breathed. But the control didn't stop there. It followed me into moments where my body simply couldn't comply, like the night I first choked on a pill. I was taught to run with an upright posture, shoulders spread wide, head held high, a stance that felt rigid and unnatural but was meant to project strength.

My body became a performance, each muscle held tight to fit their ideal. Vulnerability was forbidden, replaced with constant reminders that "only women cry."' Any softness I showed was met with disdain. They'd mutter, *Te estás portandote como una mariposa*, calling me a butterfly—a slur meant to sting, labeling me fragile, flamboyant. *Compórtate como un hombre*, they'd demand, pushing me to embody an ideal that felt impossibly far from who I was.

When my mother and sister tried to protect me, things only got worse. When they stepped in, my father would sneer, *Por qué dejas que ellas te defiendan?* (Translation: *Why do you let them defend you?*)

To him, their care wasn't kindness—it indicated my weakness by association. He saw their empathy as emasculating, a sign that I needed rescuing, and therefore wasn't strong enough to be a *real man*. Their love didn't validate me. It condemned me.

The most fragile parts of me were punished long before I could even form words around my feelings. I had just turned six. It was mid-fall, a cold evening, and I began sneezing and coughing. My mom said I was probably coming down with the flu and needed to take medicine before bed. We didn't have liquid syrup, just a few leftover pills. Swallowing pills felt impossible. Every attempt sent a wave of panic through my chest. The pill would sit in the back of my mouth like a stone, unmovable. I'd gag and try to push it down with water, but nothing worked. Four pills were wasted after I gagged and coughed the pills onto the floor, and after the third pill, my father started yelling.

He thought I was toying with them, that I was being dramatic. Then, without warning, my biological father grabbed me by the neck. "Trágatelo." ("Swallow it.")

His hand was rough, his grip tight. I could barely breathe. I tried, but the pill slipped out again. He growled, furious, and shoved another pill into my mouth. He clamped his hand over my mouth and nose, cutting off my air and choking me. I clawed at his arm, trying to signal that I couldn't breathe. My eyes watered. My chest tightened. I felt my whole body stiffen in panic. And still, he called me weak. To him, this wasn't abuse. This was training. Conditioning. Tough love. A lesson in swallowing pain—literally.

Eventually, the pill went down. Not because I learned how, but because my body gave up fighting. What lingered wasn't just the soreness in my throat or the ache in my jaw. It was the belief that my body didn't belong to me. That kindness couldn't protect me. That even the people who were supposed to love me would hurt me if I didn't perform the way they needed me to.

The darkness set in with my biological father. His approach was more violent—beatings, belittling, and brute force. His voice bore the heaviest weight, his corrections sharper, his patience thin. The pressure to meet his expectations was unrelenting.

One memory stayed buried for years. It resurfaced unexpectedly during a casual lunch with coworkers at Subway. I stepped inside and the smell of toasted bread hit me like a gut punch. My body reacted before I could name the feeling—my stomach turned, my knees nearly buckled, and I yearned to curl into a fetal position.

Karen, a kind coworker, saw my eyes watering and looked at me with concern. "Are you okay?" she asked.

I smiled weakly. "Of course. Are *you* okay?" I deflected, swallowing the memory like I had so many times before.

As a child, I had a slim frame and a small appetite—something my father couldn't tolerate. He insisted I finish a foot-long sandwich. Four bites in, I was full. But he loomed over me, eyes sharp, watching. Pressure. Demanding. His voice escalated with every bite I hesitated to take until it broke into a roar. I ate past my limits. Past comfort. Past pain. The food stretched my stomach like an overinflated balloon.

Eventually, my body revolted—I vomited. But instead of concern, he responded with disgust, not at the mess, but at *me*. He didn't check if I was okay. There was no napkin, no pause; only more shouting. "Swallow it."

Until now, I've never spoken those words out loud. That moment, that grotesque command, makes my skin crawl even now. The memory is acid—corrosive and cruel. I wasn't being punished for misbehaving. I was being punished for having needs. For having limits. As a child. And the shame? That lingered longer than the pain. It clung to me like a second skin and lodged itself in my throat.

To this day, I struggle to finish a plate of food—not because I'm full, but because fullness still feels like a threat. It wasn't just food I was forced to swallow—it was humiliation. Degradation. A message that my body wasn't mine. That I had no right to say no. That resistance equaled weakness. Every bite I took was an act of submission. But he saw even *that* as defiance. And I learned—early, painfully, permanently—that softness wasn't safe. Not even from my own body.

By the age of nine, I had internalized a truth no child should carry: I was expected to endure pain—emotional, mental, physical—without protest. At school, one teacher noticed bruises on my face and shoulders. She reported it. The school administration got involved. But when questioned, I lied and blamed my sister. I was terrified of what he'd do to me.

Feeling like I deserved it–because he had discovered I might be different–he witnessed a few classmates standing around, chatting innocently about our crushes. When it was my turn, I said, "I like Mr. Vargas." The reaction was instant—laughter, revulsion, a wall of silence. I didn't understand what I had done, only that I had violated some unspoken rule.

Their faces twisted. Their bodies recoiled. I had become something *else*. Something that is wrong. And then came the slurs: *maricón, joto, sissy, fruity*. Words that sliced deeper than any bruise.

I instinctively straightened my back, rolled my shoulders, lifted my chin, trying to wear the posture he'd beaten into me. As if standing taller could make me smaller. When I turned to leave, I saw him—my father—watching. He saw everything. And I knew at that moment I wouldn't be allowed to forget.

Eventually, Child Protective Services intervened. There was a divorce. A temporary displacement. But no comfort. No processing. No one reached out to ask how I felt. The silence from my mother, sister, and extended family said it all.

A social worker later told me, "Silence is a form of communication." What she didn't say—but I knew—was that their silence said: *You're the reason this family fell apart.*

The bullying at school didn't stop. Once I was labeled "gay," it worsened. Family visits were cold. Shame nested deep inside of me, growing like mold in dark corners. I mastered the art of performing, of pretending to be the boy they all demanded. I created masks. Wore masculinity like a costume. But beneath the armor was confusion, aching, and a constant whisper: *You don't matter. You don't belong.* That was the first time I ever conceived thoughts of not existing, being a burden, and making everyone's life easier by being gone.

I didn't choose when to come out—others did that for me. By

eighth grade, I understood more about myself, but not enough to defend myself. A friend I trusted twisted my story. A rumor spread: I had done something with a boy in the bathroom. The truth, distorted by whispers, became a weapon from a classic game of telephone. I was cornered, labeled, humiliated: *Liar. Disgusting. Homo. Faggot.*

I fled. I ran to my grandparents' house, faking a stomach ache to escape. But the pain followed. The school called. They reached my grandmother, who spoke only Spanish. I answered the phone and was instructed to bring my mother to the school. Instead, we ended up at a police station.

Detectives interrogated me in front of my mom. Five days of questions. The same ones, over and over. They believed I was covering for a teacher, a coach, some adult predator. But there was no predator. No sexual abuse. Just a story twisted into rumors. Eventually, the boy I had kissed was brought in. He denied everything. I was left alone with shame. Again.

The truth eventually surfaced, but not before I had been completely unraveled. Somewhere between the repeated interrogations and the silence that followed, I broke. I told the detectives what I hadn't dared say out loud—that I wasn't afraid of a teacher. I was afraid of what it meant to be gay in a Mexican household, for both the other boy and me—that it meant being disowned, beaten, or erased. And for a moment, they understood—more than anyone else ever had. They spoke calmly, assured the boy of his and my rights, and finally, he admitted what had happened. But by then, the damage had already sunk in with my family.

When my mother picked me up from the police station, her face didn't show relief—it wore confusion, disappointment, and something else I couldn't name back then. Before we even made it home, she looked at me with a familiar coldness and said I needed to pack my things.

I cut her off before she could finish. "I'll be emancipating myself," I said.

She scoffed, almost amused by my audacity. And then came the ridicule—not about what had happened, but about appearances. *What will people say? The neighbors? Your classmates? Their parents?* This wasn't about me—it was about her image.

At that moment, something clicked. I wasn't her child. I was her shame. And just like that, the intrusive thoughts returned, louder than before. I began to believe the unthinkable: maybe my absence would be easier for everyone.

When we arrived home, my father was waiting. Two slaps. A slur. "No son of mine will be gay."

But I stood my ground—finally. "Then you don't have a son." I walked past him—not with fear, but with something new: pride. Not the kind you inherit, but the kind you earn when you finally stop apologizing for existing. But leaving him behind wasn't the end. The war didn't end with his words—it echoed in the silence that followed. My mother, the other enforcer of shame, didn't need to raise her voice; her disapproval came through quiet glances and love that always came with conditions. That silence was its own form of violence.

Eventually, I left that house—not just in body, but in spirit. Looking back, I see now that I was dissociating, coping in all the wrong places with high school friends who masked the pain instead of healing it. In leaving, I did more than escape a home. I began the long, messy work of severing the ties between love and control, between protection and pain.

But freedom didn't come clean. The lingering thoughts stuck like thorns in my mind: *I don't belong here. I'd be better off gone.* That pain began to manifest in ways I didn't yet have the language to explain as self-harm, by nail biting, cutting. Sharp items. Burning. These were my cries for relief when words failed.

By the time I was 15, something inside me had started to fade. I couldn't focus. I was tired all the time—sometimes sleeping too much, other times not at all. I didn't feel sad exactly, just empty. Numb. Like I was drifting further away from myself. There were moments when the thought crossed my mind: *Maybe if I disappeared, all of this would finally stop.*

One day after school, I got jumped at the bus stop—words thrown like knives, shoves that turned into punches. But honestly, it wasn't just that day. It was everything. And home didn't feel any safer. That thought came back: *What if I didn't have to feel any of this anymore?*

I walked to a neighbor's house. It was quiet. Familiar. I locked the bathroom door, found something sharp, and pressed it deep into my arm, trying to let out what I couldn't say. Everything went blurry. When I opened my eyes, the door was off its hinges. My neighbor's boyfriend, Rob, had busted in. Shouting after a glimpse of Kimberly running to the phone, I begged them not to call anyone. Told them it was just from the fight. That I'd be fine. I wasn't. That day wasn't just a cry for help—it was the beginning of something I didn't yet have a name for.

Within weeks, I followed up with Kaiser Permanente and asked for help. My primary care doctor referred me to a psychologist, Dr. Gonzales. He became more than a therapist. He was a steady presence. A role model. A kind of parental figure I didn't know I needed. Through him, I learned that it was okay to seek safety. That curiosity wasn't a weakness. That I had the right to question everything—and everyone. During my sophomore year of high school, I was officially diagnosed with major depressive disorder. At the same time, I threw myself into everything I could—student government, color guard, performing arts, track, and cross-country.

I didn't have the words back then, but I would later learn I wasn't alone. The numbers confirmed what my body and heart already knew—something was deeply wrong for boys like me.

At the time, adolescent and young adult males were far less likely than females to seek help for mental health struggles. Researchers connected this to stigma, rigid expectations of masculinity, and a limited understanding of mental health (Smalley et al., 2010).

The picture was even more stark for gay, lesbian, and bisexual youth. In 2006, they reported past-year suicide attempts at nearly five times the rate of their heterosexual peers—about 21.5% compared to 4.2% (Hatzenbuehler, 2011).

Moreover, opportunity and freedom didn't come instantly—it came through grit, education, and persistently showing up for myself when others didn't. Therapy was a beacon of hope, not just for my mind but for my soul. What saved me wasn't only self-determination—it was the steady, healing presence of a male Latino therapist who gave me something I never knew I needed: space to breathe, to cry, and to learn what it truly meant to be a man outside the shadow of survival.

It was in those sessions that he introduced me to the concept of machismo—not merely as a cultural expectation, but as an inherited wound. Machismo, he explained, is a form of masculinity rooted in dominance, control, emotional suppression, and the belief that vulnerability is weakness. It's not just about how men are expected to act—it's about how generations of men were never allowed to feel. Through him, I learned I wasn't broken. I was breaking cycles of toxic masculinity.

Through grounding exercises, structured journaling, and therapy, I began to see the truth: I wasn't a fraud—I was a survivor. A boy forced to wear a mask to stay safe in a world that feared softness. But real strength? It was never in the mask unveiling; it dared to remove the mask. What I once believed was masculinity—control, silence, endurance—I've now reclaimed as something far more honest: ownership. Ownership of my emotions. My story. My truth.

Masculinity and mental health—when freed from performance—finally become real, present, and human. And isn't that the point? It was never about squeezing ourselves into their mold. It was always about shaping our own, simply because we exist. It was never about how well we fit their mold. It was always ours—because we exist and we will unapologetically and ruthlessly hold space when others ostracize us. The pain we carry doesn't always scar the skin, but it reshapes the soul. It lives in our posture, our insomnia, and our emotional absences. In anger we can't explain. In the addictions we use to cope with the aching spaces where the connection should be. They called it manhood or mental illness. But, too often, it's just survival in disguise.

So I ask you:
When did you first believe your feelings made you weak?
Who taught you that being emotional was too much?

And what part of yourself have you been forced to leave behind just to be accepted?

True healing begins when we stop pretending. When we set down the burdens that were never ours to carry and return them to the rightful owners, hold them responsible for their ignorance, misguided ways, and learned behavior. And we hope that they will hold themselves accountable for traumatizing their boys who grow up to be men.

Healing happens when we ask, " What *parts of me were silenced to make others comfortable?*

To redefine manhood is not to reject it, but to reimagine it. Manhood that welcomes softness as strength, honesty as power, and tenderness as liberation. That invites us to make space for our healing, just as my mother eventually did. With time and reflection, she had an epiphany of her own, beginning to confront the emotional wounds she had long buried. Her efforts to repair, though imperfect, reminded me that healing doesn't always come in grand gestures. Sometimes, it comes in softened eyes, fewer raised voices, and the courage to say, *I didn't know better then, but I'm trying now.*

Healing begins when we stop performing and start reclaiming. To redefine manhood is to make space for softness, for truth, for repair. For ourselves, and for the boys still learning that they're allowed to cry. The truth is: adult men in the United States make up the overwhelming majority of both victims and perpetrators of violence. Men account for 77% of suicide deaths (CDC 2023), 98% of mass shooters (Statista 2023), and nearly 90% of all homicide offenders (Bureau of Justice Statistics 2023). Men are also more likely to die in wars, to be incarcerated, and to be involved in gang-related deaths. These numbers aren't just outcomes; they're symptoms of untreated pain, social isolation, and emotional illiteracy passed down through generations.

As a sociologist and as someone who has lived this, I've come to understand that this reality isn't just about "bad decisions" or individual failure. It's about something much deeper: the ways our systems abandon boys long before they become men. It's about the weight of gender expectations, the scars of poverty, the inheritance of racial trauma, and the long shadow cast by patriarchal conditioning.

It isn't about giving up. It's about redefining what strength means. It's about challenging the lies we were taught—that to "man up" means to shut down, that "boys don't cry" means boys don't feel. This isn't surrender. It's a return. Coming home to yourself.

Healing isn't linear. It's quiet. It's messy. It's brave. It's the slow and powerful act of remembering who you were before the world told you that you weren't enough. You are not alone. You never were. And from this moment on, you don't have to stand on the sidelines of your own life.

ABOUT the AUTHOR

Eric Campos is a first-generation gay Latino writer, advocate, and social worker based in Los Angeles. He holds a double bachelor's degree in sociology and global politics and is currently pursuing a dual master's degree in social work and public health. Eric draws from his own journey—overcoming childhood trauma, addiction, and identity struggles—to tell stories that center resilience, healing, and honest dialogue. With years of experience in social work, he has supported marginalized communities through trauma-informed practices, LGBTQ+ advocacy, and rehabilitative work.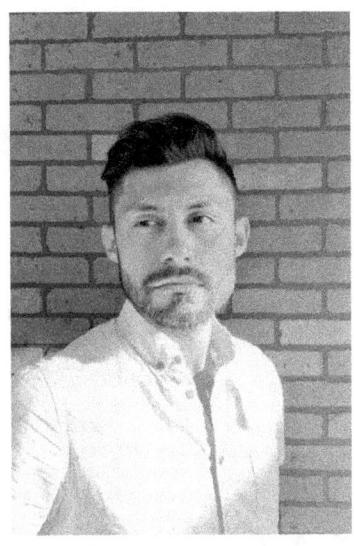

 His writing explores the hard, often unspoken parts of life, creating space for readers to confront shame and find strength in vulnerability.

Whether through his professional work or the page, Eric is dedicated to fostering change.

Social Links:
    linktr.ee/eriqeric
    @eriq.eric

Chapter 2

A Different Kind of Hard

Jason Schneider

When I turned 40, something shifted in a way I hadn't expected. My libido — once a near-constant bullhorn in the background of my life — started to quiet. At first, I welcomed it. Fewer distractions. Less compulsion. A kind of peace I hadn't known before.

From the outside, everything was good. I was single, but not lonely. I was in shape, active, and running a business I'd built from scratch. It was work that felt meaningful and aligned in a way I'd never experienced. I had meaningful friendships, work I loved, and a strong sense of self.

Which made what happened next even more disorienting.

I found myself in a moment of connection — the kind I used to long for — and nothing happened. Physically, I mean. My body didn't respond as my partner or I wanted it to. I felt confused, embarrassed, and even betrayed. And maybe the worst part... I felt alone in it.

This is not the kind of thing men talk about with each other, let alone with our partners. We joke about it, and deflect it with pills or porn or bravado. When we do hear discussions about men's sexual challenges, it's almost always framed as a mechanical failure. Just take this pill. Problem solved.

But what I was experiencing didn't feel mechanical. It felt psychological. Emotional. I wasn't sure if I was dealing with faulty hardware or the quiet, compounding weight of something deeper.

It took time, and a lot of work, to realize: it wasn't about the plumbing.

It was about pressure.

And shame.

And memory.

And the stories I'd carried quietly for years.

Growing up, sex wasn't hidden, at least not in the way it might have been for other kids. But it wasn't open in a healthy way either. I grew up through the '80s and '90s. We were latchkey kids. We had a lot of independence, not much supervision, and little to no context for the things we were experiencing. There was no internet, we just had to explore the world and sometimes found things that felt like treasures stashed in closets, garages, or under beds. For me, that meant stacks of porn magazines and VHS tapes left out by a father who struggled with sex addiction. I remember waking up in his house once to find naked strangers passed out in the living room, evidence of a sex party that I had slept through. I was maybe six years old.

Fortunately, I was being raised by my mother. She worked multiple jobs and did her best to be a positive force in my life. But my father and the culture I was growing up in weren't on her side. The media at the time, TV, movies, music, etc., portrayed a version of sexuality where men's persistence was romanticized and consent was, at best, a vague concept. Boys were expected to initiate, push, and pursue. Even when it was framed as charming or chivalrous, it was all about the pursuit.

So when I stumbled across porn at a young age, it didn't feel like a violation. It felt like a discovery. I didn't know what I was seeing, only that it was fascinating. It stirred something in me. And because no one was talking about it in a responsible way, I assumed it was mine to figure out.

I just knew that I liked what I was feeling.

And that I wasn't supposed to talk about it.

Sex, then, seemed like something people just do but don't talk about. So, at an entirely inappropriate age, I got curious. Before puberty, I had a high curiosity about sex and a fascination with bodies and sensations. I didn't know what any of it meant, only that it was powerful and compelling, and somehow mine to figure out.

But when I started acting on that curiosity ... games with friends. Silly, seemingly harmless things that kids do before they understand the rules, I got in trouble. Sometimes the other kids weren't interested. Sometimes parents were understandably upset. And I get that now. But at the time, I couldn't make sense of it. In one part of my life, at my dad's house, sex wasn't hidden. It was out in the open. Nobody talked about it in a healthy way, but it was there. It didn't feel dangerous. It felt normal.

So when the rest of my world reacted so strongly with punishment and shame, I didn't know what to feel. Slowly, a story started to build: I was bad. I was wrong. I wanted the wrong things. I wasn't aware that this was building some heavy baggage I would carry, but looking back, I can see how it shaped me. That confusion had already started to calcify into something deeper. I just didn't have the maturity or the language for it yet.

The guilt came in early and settled in deep. Even as I got older, dated, and explored, I couldn't shake the feeling that I was doing something I shouldn't. My teenage hormones didn't care, of course. I was a storm of desire, but with an undercurrent of shame that made intimacy confusing at best, and punishing at worst.

My first real girlfriend was... complicated. She pushed me into sex before I was ready, then used it regularly to manipulate me. It was used as a tool to get me to buy her things, and ditch my friends she didn't like, and it twisted me up. I learned early that sex wasn't just about bodies. It was leverage. It was power. And it could hurt.

After I left her, I started to adapt to these new lessons. Without realizing it, I became a curator of sex rather than a full participant. I studied sex, not in books or porn, but through experience and careful observation. I paid close attention to my partners' bodies, their cues, and their reactions. I learned how to read them emotionally and physically, not to manipulate, but to orchestrate. Not in a controlling or dominant way, but with the intent of creating an experience for them.

It wasn't about my orgasm. It was about theirs. About offering an experience where I was so attuned that I could disappear into the role of giver without having to wrestle with my feelings. That was the unspoken logic: if I stayed focused on their pleasure, mine couldn't be used against me. If I kept control of the encounter, I couldn't be controlled by it.

And in some ways, it worked. I felt powerful. Not a power over, but power to create something meaningful, something intimate. It gave me a sense of safety, even though it also created distance. I was physically and mentally present, but I was emotionally out of reach from my partner and from myself.

At the time, I didn't have the language to understand that. Neither did the girls I was with. We were young, connected by attraction, but without the tools to talk about what we were really experiencing. I'm sure some of them felt the disconnect. I know I did. But I didn't recognize it as loneliness. I just sensed something was missing.

It would be years before I'd understand what that something was.

Underneath the performance, I still unknowingly carried all that early shame and fear of being manipulated.

In my twenties, I leaned into serial monogamy. I thought maybe long-term relationships would bring the stability I needed to work through some of these yet-to-be-identified challenges. In some ways, they did. But I was still looking outside myself for answers. I was changing the scenario, hoping it might fix something inside myself. If I could find the right partner and the right dynamic, maybe I'd finally change. I thought I was doing the work. Showing up, trying to connect, trying to be better. But the truth is, I didn't yet know what I was avoiding.

And so, sex and the feeling of being desired served as a balm for something deeper: that I didn't really like myself. If someone else wanted me, maybe I could borrow their affection long enough to quiet the self-loathing.

My thirties were more of the same, though with shorter-term relationships. More variety. Partners from all walks of life, ages, and stories. I wasn't chasing novelty as much as I was chasing validation. The more women who wanted me, the more I could pretend I was okay. That same pattern showed up in my professional life too, as achievement, recognition, and status. Different context, same coping. The more I was wanted, the more I could pretend I was ok.

It wasn't sustainable. I could feel something starting to fray.

By the time I hit my late thirties, I knew something had to change. I wasn't ok with some of the choices I was making. I didn't want to use sex or people as a crutch anymore. I wanted connection. I wanted to build something lasting. I slowed down. Got clearer. Started looking for depth instead of distraction.

And that's when my libido began to wane.

The timing felt cruel. I was ready to approach sex differently, and my body didn't cooperate. It was frustrating, to say the least. I tried the pills, and they helped a little. But I knew there was more to what was going on. So, on the recommendation of a partner, I searched for and found a sex therapist.

In six months of work, mostly virtual, I learned more about myself than I had in decades. She helped me understand something I'd never had language for before: men deal with just as many emotional and psychological challenges around sex as women, but we don't notice them until later. Why? Because when we're younger, our libido is so strong it overrides everything else. The pressure in the pipes is so intense that it forces the water through even the most twisted and clogged plumbing.

But when the pressure of libido eases with aging, we start to notice the bends, kinks, and clogs we never noticed before. The shame. The outdated stories. The unmet needs. It all starts to matter. A lot.

Suddenly, sexual performance isn't automatic. It requires connection. Emotional spaciousness. Safety. That's what I needed — and what I had to learn how to understand and cultivate. But I also know that different men will require different things. For some, it might be about trust or different modes of stimulation. For others, it's nervous system regulation, body image, or feeling truly seen.

There's no universal formula, just a shared truth that something deeper often gets uncovered when the automatic pressure of libido fades.

And we don't usually talk about that. Not with our friends, not growing up. We never learned. We were too focused on the background bullhorn of libido.

My therapist helped me navigate all of this through a lot of work. Since I wasn't dating at the time, we focused on solo experiences. Specifically, on masturbation as a practice, not a release. That was a shift in itself. I had to unlearn the idea that it was just about getting off and start treating it as an opportunity to explore what was actually going on in my body.

We worked with my headspace. We talked about what kind of stimulation I was using and about the environment I was in. We paid attention to breath and how it shaped arousal. I'd tense up and hold it as I got closer to orgasm, and learning to breathe through those moments allowed me to be more relaxed and present. We also looked at patterns. Was I always in bed? Always in the same position? Using the same technique? What happened when I changed the setting, like music, lighting, and pace? What happened when I touched myself differently, or with more awareness?

At first, all of it felt awkward. Exposing, even though I was alone. But that was the point. I wasn't doing it to get the job done. I was doing it to understand myself better. And when something clicked, when I felt more aroused, not just physically, but on all levels, it was apparent. There was a different kind of energy. Not performative. Not pressured. Just real and grounded.

It wasn't just about orgasm. It was about relationship — with myself, with pleasure, with trust.

When I started dating again, I assumed that I'd be able to bring this newfound self-awareness into partnership. What I didn't expect was how often I'd be met with impatience.

Women will often say in articles, podcasts, surveys, and dating profiles that they want emotionally available, sexually self-aware men. Men who can be vulnerable, who've done the work, who aren't afraid to talk about intimacy or feelings. Culture tells us that this kind of man is what women are asking for.

But in practice, I often experienced something different. When I shared my story and spoke openly about sexual connection, trust, and the emotional landscape I'd been navigating, women's interest often faded. Some were kind but detached. Some just disappeared. Others got the ick. What I was offering didn't match what they seemed ready to receive.

And I get it, to a point. Women grow up in a world where male desire is constant and often threatening. Most have spent their lives navigating unwanted attention, pressure, and objectification. So they've had to develop defenses. Boundaries. Guardrails. But here's a blind spot: because women are so often the *pursued*, they're rarely asked to do the kind of intimate work they say they want men to do when paying attention to them. They haven't had to develop the same level of erotic curiosity, self-inquiry, or collaborative engagement toward men because just being a willing partner has often been enough.

That's not a criticism. It's an imbalance. And it creates a disconnect. I would approach the relationship wanting to co-create something. Not just physically, but emotionally. I wasn't looking for performance; I was looking for presence. But, more often than not, asking for something they'd never been asked to give was too much.

I don't say this with blame. I say it with sadness, and even some hope. We've built a culture that expects men to be always ready, always performing, always wanting. And when we don't show up that way, even for good, healthy reasons, we're met with confusion or disappointment.

Around our sexuality, there's more going on inside of us than we can admit or even talk about. Many of us carry shame, trauma, outdated stories, and mixed messages. Often, we don't know how deep those imprints go until the pressure eases and the faucet doesn't work when we open the valve.

That's when the work begins. Not the kind where you try harder or perform better, but the kind where you slow down and start listening to your body, your emotions, your old wiring. We learn how to untangle the twists, kinks, and clogs that quietly build up over time. The guilt we never questioned. The pressure we normalized. The habits we developed in secret.

For me, that looked like noticing when I was tensing up, holding my breath, or stuck in specific stimulation loops. I had to rewire my relationship to pleasure, not as a finish line, but as a landscape to explore. I had to examine the thoughts and feelings under the surface. The unspoken expectations, the imagined judgment, the pressure to perform. It was about shifting out of default mode and into something intentional. Not because I was trying to fix myself, but because I was finally curious about exploring more deeply.

Eventually, bringing all this awareness into connection with someone else revealed how rare it is to find someone who can meet me there. Doing this work alone is one thing. But showing up with a partner and saying, "This is where I'm at. Can we explore this together?" requires a whole new level of vulnerability.

This approach means being willing to talk through uncertainty and personal histories, to ask for patience. And it asks the same of our partners, not just to be open, but to be engaged. To co-create something meaningful. Good sex isn't about availability. It's about attunement.

That's the real work. Not pills. Not tricks. Not novelty for its own sake. It's curiosity. Presence. Self-awareness. It's doing the emotional excavation required to show up in your own body in an honest way, and inviting your partner to do the same.

This kind of intimacy takes trust. It means checking in, sharing openly, and making space for emotion and adjustment. All while trying not to overanalyze, but to stay connected. Most of us were never taught how to do that. But doing the work with yourself, a partner, or in my case, a therapist, is worth the discomfort.

If any parts of my story ring true for you, here's what I want to say to men who feel like something's wrong with them, and to the partners who love them:

There's nothing wrong with you. You're invited to dive deeper than libido-driven compulsion and into an intentional and connected sexuality.

It's uncomfortable. It's vulnerable. When we finally listen to ourselves, *really listen,* we can start building a relationship with ourselves and our partners that is more meaningful than we knew was possible.

Men's sexuality isn't a light switch. It's a whole damn complex circuit board. And it deserves the same curiosity, care, and compassion that we've come to rightfully expect from women.

We've just come to this work a little later in life.

And that's okay.

ABOUT the AUTHOR

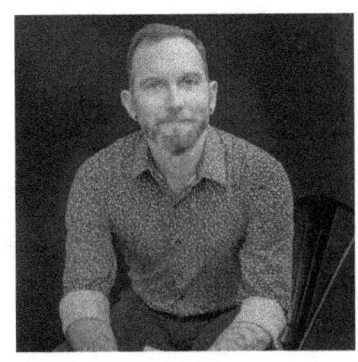

Jason Schneider is the founder of Civic Possible, a consulting firm that helps local governments and nonprofits build trust, navigate hard conversations, and create lasting change in their communities. He approaches that work in the same way he approaches life: with curiosity, humility, and a willingness to stay in the room when things get uncomfortable.

Jason grew up outside of Fresno, California, and has since called Michigan, Alaska, Oregon, Tonga, Vietnam, and Italy *home*. He's an avid climber and surfer, and currently lives in Bend, Oregon, where he's still learning what it means to live with depth, integrity, and connection — both in his work and his relationships.

This is his first time writing publicly about sexuality. It probably won't be the last.

www.civicpossible.com

Chapter 3

I Thought I Was Too Successful to be an Addict

Joshua Engle

One of the benefits of dating a doctor is that you can ask all those medical questions that you don't want to spend time seeing a doctor about. Like, *does this mole look weird?* Or, *what should I do about this headache?* Or, *do you think I'll die if I get on this airplane?*

On February 2, 2020, I woke up in Chicago with a hangover. I was living in Japan but had traveled to Chicago for First Day, a weekend for students at the University of Chicago Booth School of Business. I was certainly no stranger to hangovers. Based on how I felt, I knew I needed to throw up, hydrate, and eat some greasy food, preferably with Gatorade and a cheeseburger. It never occurred to me that knowing with that level of specificity what I needed to combat my hangover was a sign my drinking was problematic.

On this particular morning, I felt confused. I didn't think I drank that much the night before. A couple beers at the hotel bar. Four or five drinks at the official wrap-up party for First Day. Three to four more at an unofficial wrap-up party. A couple large margaritas with some late-night tacos. Ten to twelve drinks didn't seem like a lot to me, especially over the eight hours or so I was drinking. I had gone to bed thinking I had drunk more than I wanted, and certainly more than my girlfriend would have wanted. But I was actually proud of myself for not drinking more.

After I finished throwing up, I started to take stock. I had a flight that afternoon back to Japan. Breakfast was included in my stay at the hotel. I needed to pack, but I didn't have that much stuff. I traveled with Tums and Advil to take care of the nausea and headache. And then I felt a fluttering in my chest.

My pulse was high. I felt lightheaded and could feel my heart fluttering in my chest.

Uh oh. Not again.

Eleven months earlier, I had gone to the hospital with an irregular heartbeat. At the hospital, I learned it was a condition called atrial fibrillation, or AFib. Sometimes known as 'holiday heart,' AFib is the most common serious abnormal heart rhythm, affecting approximately 5% of the population. It's called holiday heart because people typically drink more at the holidays, inducing AFib. While the statistics on alcohol induced AFib aren't clear, drinking alcohol makes AFib a lot more likely. And in my case, it was directly correlated.

Unfortunately, my first bout of AFib wasn't the eye-opening experience it could have been. Sure, I had to go to the hospital and get my chest shocked to convert to a normal heart rhythm. But that didn't have anything to do with my drinking. It couldn't have anything to do with my drinking. While the 15 or so beers I had the night before were maybe a little more than I had on a typical night out, it certainly wasn't extreme. I'd had a lot more on a lot of occasions and had no need to go to the hospital. Plus, if I admitted that maybe the alcohol had played a part in it, I might have to actually do something about my drinking, and I certainly wasn't ready to acknowledge that elephant.

I was terrified and ashamed in the moment at the hospital, but afterwards, I did what any good addict does. I downplayed it. I focused on other circumstances. I ignored the medical advice of my doctor and the advice of my girlfriend, who was also a doctor. We addicts don't like people telling us anything about our consumption.

And exactly 11 months later, I found myself in the exact same situation. I knew it was AFib again. I would know that fluttering in my chest and that elevated heart rate anywhere. I faced a bit of a conundrum, though. I had a flight to catch. I needed to get back to Japan. My leave was set to expire. If I delayed my return, I'd have to tell my Navy command why. I also knew from my previous experience that, while rare, AFib can be deadly. A blood clot can form in the atria, become dislodged, and travel to the brain, causing a stroke.

So I called my girlfriend. I woke her up in the middle of the night in Japan. I shamefully told her what I was experiencing, what happened, and asked if she thought it was safe to fly. Taking a 13-hour flight back to Japan with AFib was a pipe dream at best. But I wasn't yet ready to face the truth about my problems with alcohol.

Of course, she said no. Unless I could convert on my own (unlikely, since I hadn't done so last time), I needed to get to the hospital. I went out and got some Gatorade, as the electrolytes can help. But by hotel check-out time, I was no closer to a normal sinus rhythm than I had been all morning. I called my command doctor back in Japan and let him know what was going on. I checked out of the hotel and caught an Uber to Northwestern Memorial, in downtown Chicago.

The hardest thing that happened that day wasn't the fact that the anesthesia hadn't fully set in before they shocked my chest. It wasn't the call to my girlfriend or my doctor. It wasn't even the gripping shame and self-judgment telling me I had done this to myself, that this was my fault. It was the Uber driver coming into the emergency room after he dropped me off to ask if I was contagious. He has kids at home, see, and he didn't want to get them sick.

Nope, just a fucking alcoholic, and that's not catching.

When I got back to Japan, I was presented with a choice. Knowing this had happened before, I was strongly encouraged to refer myself to the command's drug and alcohol counselor. If I chose not to refer myself, the command would be so kind as to do it for me. I was already on my way out of the Navy, but I figured a self-referral would give me more freedom to make my own decisions. If the command referred me, I wasn't sure I'd retain that freedom.

I met with the counselor, and for the first time in my life, was honest with someone about my drinking. I didn't drink in the way I thought alcoholics drank. I didn't do much morning drinking. I mostly avoided drinking during the week, unless I had the next day off. I rarely drank alone. I wasn't living under a bridge, drinking my booze out of a brown paper bag. I was a respected member of my command. I was an admiral's aide, acting as a representative for the U.S. submarine force throughout the Western Pacific. I was going to start attending the best business school in the world in the fall. How could all of that be true, and I still end up being an alcoholic?

It was a lot easier to focus on the reasons I couldn't be an addict than the reasons I could. I was never a daily drinker. I didn't wake up looking for the hair of the dog that bit me. My drinking didn't cause me to lose a job or go to jail. But I regularly drank to excess. There were many times I drove when I shouldn't have, but by the grace of God, I didn't kill myself or someone else. I blacked out a few times a month. Maybe most telling for me now, I hated sitting at home on a Friday or Saturday night when I could have been out drinking, because sitting at home meant I wasn't drinking since I was by myself.

My session with the counselor resulted in a diagnosis of severe substance use disorder. I hit eight out of the nine categories for substance abuse. The only one I missed was using every day. I was crushed. My life, as I knew it, was over. What would I do for fun, since all of my hobbies involved alcohol?

I went to the gym after my appointment in the midst of this mental spiral. Stepping into the shower after my workout was the first time I had been alone since I got my diagnosis. I burst into tears. Sobs wracked my body, and I felt an overwhelming sense of dread. This couldn't be possible. This couldn't be happening to me. Not like this. Not the disease I tried to avoid all my life.

I grew up being told I would probably be an alcoholic. With all the alcoholism on both sides of my family, my parents figured that two out of their four kids would end up struggling with addiction. My father is an alcoholic. I definitely didn't want to be like him. That's why I didn't drink every day. That's why I didn't drink by myself.

That's why I didn't drink in the morning. If I could just do everything right, control my consumption in the right way, maybe I could avoid this terrible disease and keep drinking.

All these thoughts were running through my mind as I cried alone, as quietly as I could, in the shower. All my hard work was for naught. I couldn't outrun this disease. I felt myself falling into a deep, dark hole. But from that darkness, I heard a voice in the back of my head. It delivered a message that I needed to hear. Possibly the only thing that would have given me comfort in that moment.

Sometimes the bravest thing you can do is surrender.

A sense of relief washed over my body. At that moment, I lost my desire to fight. I felt a comforting peace settle on me. I didn't fully understand what it meant then; how could surrender be brave? But I knew I had to follow that voice, that instinct.

Today, I see the bravery in that act of surrender. The cowardly route would have been to keep on going as if nothing had happened, as if nothing had changed. I could have kept my head stuck in the sand and continued with the life I was comfortable with. Or I could surrender to the moment. I could surrender to my diagnosis. I could accept that life, as I knew it, was over. I could do the brave thing and work to build a new life from the ashes of the old. Nothing would be the same, and that was terrifying. But in the face of the fear, I was able to be brave.

I accepted that I had a problem with alcohol that day. It seemed obvious in retrospect. However, I wasn't ready to admit I was an alcoholic yet. I stopped drinking at that point and haven't had a drink since. By the time I got to rehab at an in-person treatment center a few months later, I had some sober time under my belt. Sober time can be dangerous for an addict. I had weathered the onset of the COVID-19 pandemic without drinking. I had booze in my apartment until I moved out to head back stateside, and I didn't drink it. More reasons I looked at to prove to myself and anyone who would listen that, while I was a problem drinker, I certainly wasn't an alcoholic.

At rehab, I was introduced to the Big Book of Alcoholics Anonymous. When I read through it for the first time, I thought, *wow, these folks have a real problem. I'm glad I'm not like them.*

It wasn't until a few weeks later that the reality really set in for me. I knew I could say *no* to the next drink. I had kept myself from drinking for four months before I arrived at treatment. I was pretty sure I could say no to the drink after the next one. But what dawned on me was that there was some drink, somewhere down the line, that I wasn't sure I could say *no* to. For me, to drink is to risk death. Not just in the typical sense of an addict ending up in jails, in institutions, or dead. Any time I drink, I risk a recurrence of AFib. Any recurrence of AFib could lead to a stroke. The odds of a drink causing AFib and a stroke are small. But the fact that I couldn't definitively say that I wouldn't pick up a drink when a drink could fucking kill me rocked my world.

It was easy to stay on the straight and narrow, saying all the right things in rehab. The structure and support made sure of it. Afterwards, recovery didn't come easy to me. I struggled to truly see myself as someone battling the disease of addiction. That fall, I started at Chicago Booth, U.S. News's top-ranked MBA program. Addicts lose jobs to their addictions. Addicts get DUIs or go to prison. Addicts don't get into business school. Addicts don't have successful careers in the military.

Plus, all my new friends in business school were drinking and partying with impunity. I was like them, wasn't I? They didn't have to spend their free time going to meetings, talking to other addicts and alcoholics. Why should I? I started drifting away from the recovery community. I truly believed I could keep myself sober, and I didn't think the one meeting a week I was attending was making much of a difference in my life, anyway.

That fall, I experienced the deepest depression of my life. I was isolated in a new city. I was making new friends, but I felt disconnected from the world around me. I no longer had my friend and companion, alcohol. I coped with porn, ice cream, and isolation instead. I struggled to adjust to a new life without my old coping mechanism. But slowly, through the help of therapy and medication, I started to climb out of it. Started to feel like myself again.

I can't say for sure how my story would have played out if I hadn't drifted away from recovery. Maybe I would have developed other tools to manage my depression and anxiety earlier. Maybe I would have weathered the storm better and stayed sober. It's impossible to know, but I think I needed to have the experiences I had to get to where I am today. I had already started planting seeds in rehab.

Around the midway point of my time in rehab, I'd asked my therapist what he thought about me smoking weed. People kept telling me that if I used drugs, it would take me back to drinking, but that didn't seem likely. See, I had accepted myself as an *alcoholic*, but I had never mixed the two. So I wouldn't have the mental association of getting high and getting drunk. I think I mentally relapsed when my therapist told me it would probably be alright as long as I kept it to a couple of times a week. That was all the permission I needed.

I was a smart alcoholic, though. I knew there was some danger in it. So I figured a period of sobriety would make it alright. I would wait until I had a year of sobriety, and if I still wanted to smoke weed then I could probably do so safely. I didn't do it right away. I waited a little bit. I think I started with edibles on a spring break trip. But once I got started, I was off to the races.

I've never been one for moderation. I tried to keep it to once or twice a week, like my therapist recommended. For the first few weeks, I managed it. But it wasn't long before I started using it every evening to unwind. But soon, that wasn't enough. I started wanting it earlier and earlier in the day. I started rushing through my school work so I could start smoking. After a while, I didn't even wait for that. It would light up mid–, telling myself that the weed made me more creative, that I would be better at my work while I was high. But most of the time, I got too high to do any actual work.

Six months in or so, I started wondering if this was a problem. I was smoking every day, earlier and earlier in the day. But I wanted to keep going. I started trying to create rules for myself around my smoking. I had to put all my paraphernalia away before I went to bed, so I wouldn't be tempted in the morning by the last bit of a joint. I went back to finishing my work before I started smoking.

All these rules were like the attempts I had made in the past to control my drinking. *I'll only drink beer tonight—or only wine. I won't drink on weeknights. I won't drink in the morning. I'll go out tonight, but I won't do shots.* Or, *I'll go out, but I won't drink* (which never worked for me). The rules were different, but the cause was the same: I couldn't handle my substance.

Over time, I came to realize that it was an actual problem for me. One moment stands out in my memory. I was having a fight with my girlfriend. I couldn't tell you what the argument was about now, and I doubt I could have articulated it then. But as we were arguing on the phone, I lit up a joint. All of a sudden, the issue didn't seem that bad. I completely stopped arguing and let it go. And I realized that it had never been about the argument or my girlfriend. It had everything to do with the fact that I hadn't smoked all day and was jonesing.

Sometime after that, I decided to take a break. I was nearing the end of my time in grad school and wanted to make the most of it. I decided I would take the last quarter off from smoking so I could be more present. I went on spring break with my girlfriend, and I planned not to smoke until after graduation when I got back. Once I got home, however, I realized that there was still some weed in my apartment, and technically, the spring quarter hadn't started yet. I could finish up what I had and **then** stop. Three or four days later, I was on my way to the dispensary again. I rationalized it somehow. I remember being on the phone with my girlfriend, who knew I had intended to take the last quarter off, rationalizing my trip to the dispensary.

Eventually, that quarter, I did stop. I gave all my paraphernalia to a friend so that I wouldn't have any opportunity to smoke. Life got better without smoking all the time (surprise, surprise), but I still wasn't where I wanted to be. I kept searching for what would help. I tried quitting all stimulants (prescription and coffee) cold turkey. That didn't help. It just made me tired and annoyed my girlfriend. I read a lot of self-development books. And for some reason, everything I read kept bringing me back to 12 step programs. I tried reading Russell

Brand's book, *Recovery*. Turns out it's all about the 12 steps. I read *Healing the Shame That Binds You*, thinking I could heal my shame and feel better. But that book ended up being about how the 12 steps help heal your shame.

Eventually, a couple of weeks after the girlfriend and I broke up, and I was feeling miserable, I decided to try 12-step recovery again. *Could all these people be wrong? Maybe it could work for me this time around.* And it did.

I showed up to meetings. I connected with other alcoholics and addicts. I followed suggestions to create community by calling other men every day. I learned to pray and explore what a relationship with a Higher Power, personal to me, could look like. And my life got better. Not immediately. But over time, the angst I felt most of my life started to slip away. The uncomfortable feelings I would get around other people, in crowded settings, didn't feel so unbearable. I was able to, for maybe the first time in my life, take myself out of the equation and not take everything so damn personally all the time.

My entire life has changed twice already since I came back into 12 step recovery. When I came back, I was living at my parents' house in Chicago, searching for a job after graduating from business school. Eventually, I found a job that took me to Washington, D.C. I left that job after 15 months to become a life coach, and left D.C. six months later to become a digital nomad.

I couldn't even imagine the life I have today before I quit drinking in February 2020, or even when I quit smoking weed in August 2022. My world and the possibilities in it continue to grow. And I expect I can't even imagine what will be possible for me in the years to come. I still have temptations from time to time. I'll be walking through a grocery store and think that a glass of wine with dinner sounds nice. Or I'll walk through a park and catch a hint of weed, and take a deeper breath. But I recognize those ideas for what they are: signs of my addiction. As I travel around the world, I'm able to find 12 step recovery everywhere I go. If I happen upon a place where I can't find an in-person, English-speaking meeting, I can hop on Zoom anytime, day or night. There's always a meeting going on somewhere in the world. And if I have cultivated a community of fellows, I can call anytime for support, alcohol and drug-related, or otherwise.

My calling as a coach has given me a mission, to help men become better men, and a purpose, to be a vessel for my Higher Power's will in the world. I'm able to support other men (and women) on their path to finding and creating the life that they truly desire. For so long, I pursued the life that I thought other people wanted for me or would look on favorably. But now, I pursue a life that's uniquely meaningful to me, and I support my clients in doing the same.

I've been able to create the life that I want through coaching. But first and foremost, in all the best things in my life, is the foundation I've built through sobriety and recovery.

ABOUT the AUTHOR

Joshua Engle is a leadership and life coach who helps high-achieving men navigate the gap between external success and internal fulfillment. A 2012 U.S. Naval Academy graduate, he served eight years as a submarine officer before earning his MBA from Chicago Booth in 2022 and transitioning to coaching.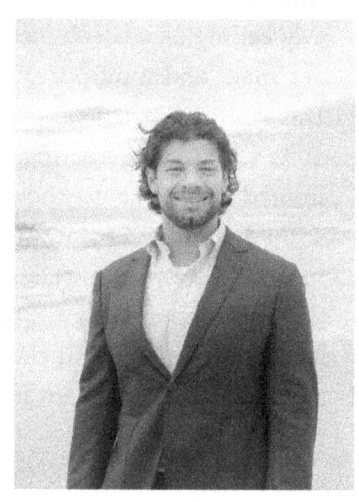

Despite achieving conventional markers of success throughout his military and business career, Joshua struggled with addiction—a reality that challenged his perceptions of what addiction looks like. He began his recovery journey in 2020, and his story explores how external achievement can coexist with internal struggle.

As a graduate of Accomplishment Coaching's 12-month program, he brings a strategic, holistic approach to his practice at Engle Coaching. He sponsors other men in 12-step recovery and writes about masculine development and personal growth through his Substack and Instagram. He's currently writing a book exploring masculine archetypes through modern pop culture. Based in Chicago, he's traveling throughout Latin America as a digital nomad, continuing to explore what authentic success means.

Social Links:
www.instagram.com/joshuaenglecoach/
joshuaengle.substack.com/

Chapter 4

The Hidden Determinants

How Love, Connection, and Vulnerability Shape a Man's Mental Health

Coach Zeke

Beneath the armor of every strong man lies a heart that aches for connection. For every man who's ever been told to "toughen up," this chapter is for you. In a world that praises stoicism and quiet endurance, the emotional battles of men are often waged in silence. We've been taught that strength means withholding, that resilience means carrying on without complaint, and that vulnerability is a weakness to be avoided at all costs. And as men, we've been taught to wear these expectations as a "badge of honor."

But what if the opposite is true? What if our mental health is not determined by how much we can endure alone, but by how deeply we can connect to ourselves, to others, and to the world around us?

In the pages that follow, I invite you to strip away the layers of pretense and lean into the uncomfortable, yet liberating, act of being fully known. We will explore the transformative power of love, the vital need for connection, and the often-overlooked strength in vulnerability. I want you to look beyond the surface and into the spaces where real growth and healing happen – the places where we learn to trust, to love, and to reveal the parts of ourselves we've been taught to hide.

Because the strongest men are often the quietest, not because they lack words, but because they've been taught to swallow them. It's time to change that. It's time to unlearn the silence and embrace the truth that real power lies in being deeply human.

The Silent Struggle: Unpacking the Male Emotional Blueprint

From a young age, boys are taught the "rules". Be tough. Don't cry. Don't talk too much about your feelings. And whatever you do, never show weakness. These lessons aren't always spoken outright. Sometimes they're absorbed from a father's stoic silence, a coach's reprimand, or a peer group that polices emotion like it's a crime. But make no mistake: the emotional blueprint handed to most men is forged in silence and suffering, and often enforced through shame.

That silence becomes armor. And that armor gets heavy.

As men age, the emotional suppression that once felt like strength begins to corrode from the inside. Studies confirm this truth. The American Foundation for Suicide Prevention reports that men die by suicide at a rate nearly four times higher than women.[1] Yet men are far less likely to seek therapy or speak openly about emotional distress. Not because they *feel* less, but because they've been taught to feel *less publicly*.

So we don't just suffer in silence—we suffer *because* of it.

Here's the paradox: the very behaviors society calls *manly*—emotional stoicism, self-reliance, invulnerability—are the same behaviors most closely linked to poor mental health outcomes. According to a 2015 study published in *Psychology of Men & Masculinity*, men who strongly adhere to traditional masculine norms experience higher levels of psychological distress, depressive symptoms, and suicidal ideation.[2]

But this chapter isn't about blaming anyone for the systems that shaped us. It's about breaking the spell. About seeing the silence for what it is: an outdated inheritance we no longer need to carry. This chapter is also about cultivating a new *prism* through which all men can view their experiences. A prism that allows for being human unapologetically.

Because buried beneath the tough exterior lies an entire world of unmet mental and emotional needs—a longing to be fully acknowledged, to be seen at our deepest levels, to be loved without needing to measure up to an unhealthy, if not impossible standard. Men don't lack emotional depth. Many are drowning in it. They just haven't been given the tools—or permission—to name it.

There is strength in the man who knows he needs love. There is wisdom in the one who reaches for connection. These aren't signs of weakness—they are signs that you're still alive, still human, and still whole beneath it all.

The Mask Nearly Broke Me

This isn't just theory. I've lived it.

It was around Christmas in 2016. My business was struggling, and the financial strain was crushing. As a single dad, I was battling to provide for my kids. The pressure of being the first son in a Nigerian family weighed heavily on me. Years ago, my father had passed away, and I felt an immense responsibility to uphold my family and fulfill my expected role. But as the business stumbled, no one knew that I felt like I was failing on every front.

Instead of receiving support, I was met with blame and judgment from those around me. My family, rather than offering a shoulder to lean on, pointed fingers. You see, unknowingly, they too were subject to the thoughts and expectations they were taught by our culture and society. Those expectations to be the unwavering pillar of strength had turned into a crushing weight.

This lack of support pushed me into the deepest depression I'd ever known. It wasn't just emotional; it was logical, which was the scariest part. In my mind, I was convinced the world would be better off without me, and that my family would be relieved of a burden. I rationalized that my family would mourn me for a bit, but in the end, would rebound and be better off without me. It was a terrifyingly dark place, and I found myself planning how to exit this world quietly, convinced it was the most rational solution. I felt like I was standing at the edge of an abyss. Far too close to the edge. I was catching a glimpse of how fleeting mental health can be.

What pulled me back was a conversation with my daughter, Jordan, who was only nine at the time. I asked her if she thought people would miss me if I were gone. With the pure innocence and honesty of a child, she told me how much I mattered, how much my presence meant to her. That moment shattered the illusion that I was a burden. It was the love of my daughter that saved me, and that conversation was the first step on my journey back to myself.

Eventually, with the support of Jordan and her mother, I emerged from that darkness. But that depression had been fueled by the unreasonable standards of masculinity and the lack of understanding from those who could have been my safety net.

That was the moment I realized that true strength isn't about living up to a rigid archetype. And it isn't about carrying the weight of the world on your shoulders. You simply don't win any awards or medals for how much burden you can carry alone.

I learned that true strength is also shown by embracing love, connection, and vulnerability—and finding the courage to rewrite the narrative.

The Power of Love: The Foundation of All Mental and Emotional Health

Love is often portrayed as a soft emotion, something antithetical to a man's purpose. Yet, for men and everyone else, love is more than just an emotion—it's a foundational pillar of mental and emotional health and resilience. It's the force that grounds us, connects us, and gives our very lives meaning.

Redefining Love in Masculinity

Traditionally, men have been conditioned to view love as vulnerability —a weakness that compromises their strength. They have been taught *not* to lean into love as an answer, almost ever. But real love, practiced fully and without fear, is not weakness. In fact, it is a deeply masculine act. It demands presence, courage, and devotion. When a man opens himself to love, he does not lose power—he steps into it more fully.

In my upcoming book, *The Many Great Loves of Superman*, I explore the practical and metaphysical nature of love—how the energy of love is the catalyst for all joy and peace, how it transforms our relationship to the world, and especially our relationship with ourselves. Love is absolutely necessary for mental health—not just for women, not just for children—but for men. *Especially* for men.

Because the truth is, we are not built to do this thing called life alone. We are wired for love. And without it, a man may appear composed on the outside, but he can be crumbling internally without purpose, disconnected, disoriented, and quietly depleted.

The Science of Love and Well-being

Science agrees. *The Harvard Study of Adult Development,* an 80+-year study on happiness and longevity, concluded something beautifully simple: "Good relationships keep us happier and healthier. Period."[3] Men who reported strong, loving relationships were not only more likely to avoid depression, but they also lived longer and retained sharper cognitive function in their later years. Love wasn't a bonus—it was actually the backbone of a healthy life.

The Healing Power of Everyday Love

Love doesn't always come in grand gestures. Sometimes it's the way your partner greets you at the door with a warm smile after a brutal day. It's the child who throws their arms around you without needing a reason. It's the softness of home—the laughter, the shared meal, the silent embrace that says, *you're safe here… you won't be judged… I won't point fingers… I am here to love you.*

I've seen it in my own life. I've felt drained from the world's weight, worn down from more battles than I could name, but a single moment of real love—a conversation, a hug, or a soft voice that reminded me who I am—restored my soul. Those moments remind me that I'm far from broken. I'm just a man who needed a reminder, needed his purpose, a man who needed love.

That's the power of love: it reminds us that we're not alone. It gives us the strength to keep going. And gives all the reasons to endure.

Connection: The Antidote to Isolation

In a world that often equates masculinity with self-reliance, many men find themselves navigating life's challenges in solitude. The silent expectation to "man up" and handle problems alone has led to an epidemic of isolation among men, with profound implications for mental health.

The Crisis of Disconnection

Recent studies highlight a troubling trend: young American men are experiencing unprecedented levels of loneliness. A Gallup poll conducted between 2023 and 2024 revealed that 25% of U.S. men aged 15 to 34 reported feeling lonely frequently during the previous day. This isolation isn't just a fleeting emotion; it's a significant health risk. The World Health Organization equates the health risks of chronic loneliness to smoking 15 cigarettes a day.

The roots of this disconnection are multifaceted. Societal norms have long discouraged men from expressing vulnerability or seeking emotional support. From a young age, boys are often taught to suppress their feelings, leading to emotional repression and a reluctance to form deep, meaningful connections. Even worse, as a result of this conditioning from childhood, the natural communicative tools that children use to foster genuine communication are not even "sharpened' due to a lack of use. This leaves men in a position where even when they realize they need, or want, more connection in their lives, they often don't know how to go about it. In turn, this manifests an awkwardness around creating connection, which then leads to a palpable feeling of "self-consciousness" when attempting to connect. The end result is the behavior of actively not connecting with those around them for fear of judgment from themselves subconsciously, and others outwardly. In short, this can be a vicious cycle. This cultural conditioning fosters a sense of alienation, even within close relationships.

The Healing Power of Connection

Connection is not a luxury; it's a necessity. Human beings are inherently social creatures, and meaningful relationships are vital for emotional well-being. Connection to others is, in fact, among the primary ways we learn and grow as human beings. For men, fostering connections can serve as a powerful antidote to the isolation that so often accompanies traditional masculine roles.

How do we remedy the problem of isolation among men?

My first answer is quite simple. However, we ALL have a role to play in this. First, we must normalize the concept of men being expressive, and it must start at an early age. When I say this, I am not referring to only sharing their emotions. We need to encourage the sharing of thoughts and perspectives on all things. Consider the "ripple effect" of an action such as asking a child a philosophical question about their feelings or coping mechanisms, or better yet, asking a group of children the question. Things like this often are the spark that lights the fire of authentic connection. We begin to notice the similarities within all of us. I contend that nothing creates a connection more than seeing ourselves in each other. I even hypothesize that if we practiced this single exercise in communication, most of the troubles of the world would be solved.

But that's another conversation, for another book...lol.

My next answer, well, I'm speaking to my brothers directly on this one: we also need to normalize making the time for, being actively present in, and holding the sacred space for us men, to share with one another. Why? Well, because who can understand the plight of a man better than... well... a man. It is hard being a woman. Let me state this first for our queens out there. But... allow me to say: It is damn hard being a man, as well. We know this. We feel it every day. Thus, we also know that we can understand that journey and plight in ways that our wives, sisters, mothers, and daughters may not be able to fully grasp. So I invite my kin, men, to be our own healers and create spaces for ourselves to congregate and connect on a deep and meaningful level.

Other ways to foster connection can include the simple act of sharing a meal with a friend, engaging in a heartfelt conversation, or participating in community groups. These interactions provide a sense of belonging and affirmation, reminding men that they are not alone in their struggles. Initiatives like Andy's Man Club in the U.K. have recognized this need, offering peer-to-peer support groups where men can openly discuss their mental health challenges in a safe, non-judgmental environment.

Remembering Humanhood, Reclaiming Brotherhood, Rebuilding Wholeness

The truth is, connection isn't just a remedy—it's a reclamation. When men begin to reconnect with themselves, with each other, and with their communities, we don't just feel better. We *become whole again*. We remember that strength was never meant to be a solo act. Real strength includes the courage to be seen, the humility to be held, and the wisdom to know we are *not meant to do this life alone.*

It's time we shed the armor of isolation and pick up something far more powerful: *authentic connection.* The kind where we don't have to perform, pretend, or posture. The kind where we are safe to tell the truth, feel deeply, and still be respected as powerful, capable men.

And while the road to deep connection might feel unfamiliar at first, it's paved with simple, everyday choices, like checking in on a friend, opening up at a men's circle, mentoring a younger brother, listening without fixing, or just being fully present. These small acts are *sacred*. They are seeds that grow into belonging, resilience, and healing, not just for you, but for others as well.

So to my brothers reading this: your heart is not a liability—it's a compass. Let it guide you back to the tribe you've been missing. Let it remind you that connection isn't a weakness. It's a superpower. And it is, indeed, the medicine the world—and your soul—has been waiting for.

Practical Steps to Reconnect

An important note is that building and rebuilding connections requires intentional effort. Here are some practical steps men can take to foster meaningful relationships:

- **Reach Out**: Make a conscious effort to connect with friends or family members. A simple phone call or message can rekindle relationships that have lapsed over time.
- **Join a Group**: Participate in community groups or clubs that align with your interests. Shared activities provide a natural setting for forming new friendships.
- **Seek Support**: Don't hesitate to seek professional help or join support groups. Engaging with others facing similar challenges can provide comfort and perspective.
- **Practice Being Vulnerable**: Allow yourself to express emotions and share personal experiences. Vulnerability fosters deeper and more authentic connections and mutual understanding.

Vulnerability – The Secret Gateway to Authentic Strength

Vulnerability is often misunderstood, especially by men. We've been conditioned to see it as exposure, as weakness, as something to avoid or hide behind closed doors. However, true vulnerability isn't the absence of strength, but it can certainly be the birthplace of it. When a man allows himself to be seen, fully and honestly, he taps into a power that is divine in its making. The power to touch anyone and everyone deeply.

The Masculine Myth Around Vulnerability

Let's be honest: most men have been raised in environments where vulnerability is punished—socially, emotionally, sometimes even physically. We've been trained to keep it in, suck it up, and push forward. Crying was for the girls. Talking about our pain was "soft." But this cultural script has a cost—and it's a steep one.

The American Psychological Association has documented that restrictive emotionality—one of the key components of traditional masculine ideology—is a significant predictor of mental health struggles, including depression and anxiety.[3] Men who avoid emotional expression are more likely to experience internalized stress, breakdowns in relationships, and emotional burnout.

The irony? Vulnerability is the very thing that could have saved them.

Vulnerability as Power

When a man owns his emotions instead of suppressing them, when he admits he's struggling instead of pretending he's not, he sends a message to his subconscious, first and most importantly. Then, silently, to the world as a byproduct.

Vulnerability says: *I trust myself enough to reveal what's real.*

It says: *I am worthy of love, even in my brokenness.*

It says: *I am still masculine, even while being inexorably human.*

Most importantly, it says: *And that's okay.*

Here's what's beautiful: vulnerability doesn't just make *you* stronger. It strengthens everyone around you. It gives your sons permission to feel. It shows your daughter that sensitivity and strength can live within the same man. It teaches your partner how to love you better. Vulnerability isn't self-indulgence—it's often the best that leadership has to offer.

Say this next part out loud with me.

Every human being, at their core, carries two sacred desires:

First, to be exactly who they are—heart, soul, flaws, gifts, and all.

And secondly, but so often overlooked, they desire to be genuinely loved for being that exact version of themselves.

But here's the paradox: we can never be *loved* for who we truly are if we don't have the courage to *show* who we truly are. Vulnerability is the bridge, and the ONLY bridge, I might add, between those two human needs.

If a man hides his pain, his tenderness, his truth, then even if love shows up at his door, it won't "know" him because he hasn't allowed the world to see *him* yet. Only a projection. Only the armor.

The love we all deeply crave can only find us when we stop hiding.

When a man finally says, "This is me. Not the image. Not the performance. Just *me*," something sacred happens:

He gives himself the opportunity to love *himself* fully. He gives others the opportunity to love him fully, as well. And more than that, he gives *himself* the chance to experience the kind of love that actually heals.

What Vulnerability Looks Like in Real Life

It's the father who finally opens up about how lost he felt after his own father died.

It's the husband who tells his wife, "I'm scared, and I need your help."

It's the man who says to his brother, "I miss you," even though they haven't said those words since they were kids.

It's showing up. Speaking honestly. Taking off the mask—if only for a moment—and letting someone see what's underneath.

Think of this for a second: how happy, self-assured, motivated, and excited would you be if you knew the world would accept you *exactly* as you are? Can you imagine being depressed, insecure, or lacking confidence under those circumstances? I, for one, cannot. But here's the kicker: *how can you be accepted and loved for who you are without the vulnerability to actually show who you are?*

The Truth is Sexy

Some time ago, back when I was in high school, I coined the phrase *The truth is sexy*. At the time, it was a response to a corny pick-up line that a friend of mine said to a lady he was interested in. I had always believed pick-up lines to be ridiculously silly. Mainly because I've always felt this inner knowing that inauthenticity is always easily felt by our fellow human beings. And yes, I'm saying it, pick-up lines are inauthentic and corny. But, this works both ways; authenticity, also, is typically felt intrinsically by people, as well. And authenticity is birthed through–you guessed it–vulnerability. Being vulnerable enough to show your family, friends, romantic partner, and the world exactly who you are is a game-changer that leads to connection and ultimately love. And mark my words, the vast majority of the world will celebrate that courage, that authenticity, and that vulnerability. The truth–*your* truth–will always be sexy.

Integrative Practices: Exercises for Inner Work

Purpose: bring love, connection, and vulnerability into your daily life

True transformation doesn't come from reading alone, but from *living* the truths we uncover. Love, connection, and vulnerability are not concepts reserved for deep conversations or rare breakthroughs. They are daily practices. Embodied rituals. Lived experiences.

As men, many of us have learned to *do* rather than *feel*. These integrative exercises are not about becoming someone new—they're about removing the barriers to who you already are. A man capable of deep love. A man wired for connection. A man courageous enough to be vulnerable.

These practices are designed to help you internalize the work of this chapter, not just intellectually, but somatically, emotionally, and spiritually. If done with intention, these small moments of truth can change everything.

Exercise 1: For Love – Reclaiming the Heart

Title: *The Love Inventory*
Instructions:

1. In a journal or notebook, make two columns. On the left, list every person in your life that you love deeply—from family, to friends, to mentors, to spiritual figures.
2. On the right, answer the following for each person:
   - When was the last time I told them I love them?
   - Do they know why I love them?
   - How often do I show it in a way they receive?

Reflect: What would shift if I expressed love more freely and more often?

Purpose: This exercise helps reignite your heart space. Many men feel love deeply but express it rarely. Reclaiming this expression can create healing not just in you, but in the people around you.

Exercise 2: For Connection – Creating Sacred Presence

Title: *The 5-Minute Presence Practice*
Instructions:

1. Choose one person each day to give your full, undivided attention to for five minutes—no phone, no TV, no multitasking.
2. Ask them a real question: "How are you really feeling today?"
3. Listen with your entire body. Don't fix. Don't solve. Just *witness*.

Purpose: Connection is built in presence, not performance. This daily ritual cultivates depth, empathy, and emotional intelligence. It reminds both you and the other person that *they* matter, and that *you* do, too.

Exercise 3: For Vulnerability – Releasing the Mask

Title: *The Emotional Debrief*
Instructions: At the end of the day, take five minutes to reflect on the following prompts:

1. Where did I feel something deeply today, but kept it inside?
2. Where did I share something honest about myself?
3. Did I avoid vulnerability out of fear? If so, what was I afraid of?

You can journal these, speak them into a voice note, or share them with a trusted person.

Purpose: This exercise helps normalize vulnerability as a daily practice. Like a muscle, your capacity to show up as your full self strengthens with use.

Group or Interactive Exercise: Building Brotherhood

Title: *The Circle of Truth*
Instructions:

1. Gather a group of men—this can be friends, colleagues, or part of a support circle.
2. Sit in a circle and go around, one by one. Each man shares:
   - One area in his life where he feels emotionally stuck
   - One fear he hasn't yet named
   - One truth he wants to begin living
3. No one interrupts, advises, or corrects. The only response allowed is: "Thank you for sharing that."

Purpose: This exercise builds emotional safety, brotherhood, and mutual respect. It teaches men that vulnerability does not weaken them—it *awakens* them.

Review and Implementation

You've taken a short journey through some of the most powerful forces in the human experience. You've explored how love heals, how connection strengthens, and how vulnerability liberates. These are not feminine traits. They are *human* ones. And they are part of your design as a man.

What's next is simple: don't just *understand* it—*live it.*

The Path Forward: Embracing a New Narrative

This chapter hasn't been about *changing* who you are. It's about *returning* to who you've always been.

Underneath the armor, beyond the roles and expectations, is a man —fully human—who was born with the capacity to love deeply, to connect meaningfully, and to express himself without shame. That man is not broken. He's not weak. He's not too emotional or not emotional enough. He's whole. He's powerful. He's *you*.

We were never meant to do this alone. And we certainly weren't meant to suffer in silence. The path forward is not about perfection, but about permission—the permission to feel, to speak, to soften, to seek help, to show up raw and real and still be worthy of love.

We heal through love.

We rise through connection.

We lead through vulnerability.

The old model of masculinity told us to dominate, to endure, to never show cracks. But cracks let the light in. And when you embrace the light of who you truly are, you give others permission to do the same.

This is your invitation to start living unmasked. Not for anyone else—but for yourself. Because you matter. Because your truth matters. Because the world doesn't need more perfectly composed men—it needs more *whole* ones.

So take what you've discovered here—about love, connection, and vulnerability—and let it become a new way of being. Let it reshape your relationships. Let it rewire your self-worth. Let it heal your wounds and scars. And let it be the substance that your mental health is built upon, not in theory, but in action.

Because the strongest man in the room is not the one who hides it all. It's the one who knows he doesn't have to anymore.

ABOUT the AUTHOR

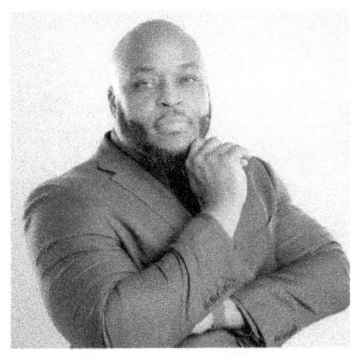

Azuka Tuke, known to many as Coach Zeke, is a transformational keynote speaker, master-level life coach, fitness and nutrition expert, and the visionary founder of Coach Zeke Amplified. With over two decades of experience helping individuals unlock their full potential, Azuka brings a powerful blend of science-backed strategy and soul-level wisdom to every space he enters. His work is rooted in holistic well-being—physical, mental, emotional, and spiritual—and grounded in one core principle: love heals everything.

He is the author of **The Many Great Loves of Superman**, in which, through "love letters" and "love lessons," he shares intimate stories and metaphysical insights on the nature of love, human consciousness, and personal evolution.

Through his keynotes, coaching, and content, Coach Zeke continues to be a catalyst for emotional freedom and mastery, authentic living, and the reclamation of masculine wholeness.

To connect with him and/or explore his programs, visit CoachZekeAmplified.com or reach out directly at CoachZekeAmplified@gmail.com.

Or use this QR Code to join "The Many Great Loves Of Superman" book community on Telegram at
t.me/+oNls1NGmgy8xZjYx

Chapter 5

What, Mental Health?

Juan Camilo Posada Arenas

Twenty years ago, if you had asked me what mental health was, I probably would've said it was some kind of vitamin or an opioid you took for a headache. Back then, my life context was completely different, and health—whether physical or mental—wasn't even on my radar.

I want to be very honest and open with my story. At age 15, my mother decided to separate from my father, and due to financial issues, we moved to what was then considered the most dangerous neighborhood—or "comuna"—in all of Latin America: the infamous Comuna 13 in Medellin, Colombia.

If you've never heard of it, it's very similar to the favelas in Rio, Brazil—houses stacked on top of each other along steep hillsides accessible only by stairs. It was the setting for the notorious Operación Orión, a military campaign aimed at dismantling paramilitary violence. I'm no political expert, and I don't want to sway your opinion, but what I can tell you is that it was a dark chapter in the city's history. I remember seeing international magazine covers that read "Medellin: The Most Dangerous City In the World." Between that global perception and the Hollywood movies that portrayed my city as a jungle, many versions of Comuna 13 emerged—but I didn't live in the heart of it.

Technically, the comuna is a politically defined quadrant, and each one is massive. I lived in an open housing unit, not in the slums directly, so we weren't in danger, but hearing gunshots was common, and danger was always an option if you chose to go down that road.

My family and I were all about appearances. We lived in a middle-class area, but after my father's three bankruptcies, abundance and safety were not part of our daily conversations. There were months with no power, no water, and due to my parents' conflicts, it was we—the kids—who suffered the most. That was one of the main reasons for the separation and why my mother had to move to a place where every so-called friend and family member abandoned her.

At 15, I didn't fully understand what was going on, but I started taking on responsibilities I wasn't ready for—fatherly, provider roles that stripped me of my childhood. And just like that, without warning, my first identity crisis—and my first mental health crisis—began.

It was a tough time. Sometimes there wasn't enough food, and my mother would ask the church priest for groceries. She had to borrow money for bus fare, and I inherited a heavy, rusty pink bike that trained me to sweat and built an unbreakable character. We were in survival mode. And when you're surviving, everything else comes second. You're just trying to get by with the basics.

I'm not here to romanticize anything. Honestly, at the time, it didn't feel that bad. I could still go to school, play sports, drink a beer—even if it meant choosing between that and the bus fare home from the hangout spot, La Villa. I often chose to walk, and I don't regret it.

But now, as an adult, talking with my siblings and mom, I realize that she lived in constant scarcity and stress—something that still shows up in her life today. And I'm sure, even if I didn't know it then, I absorbed all of that. It shaped my relationship with money, abundance, mental health, and peace.

Not long ago, I heard 50 Cent say, "Depression is a luxury you can afford when your life is good." And yes, when you're just trying to survive, you don't have time to be depressed. Your priorities are food, shelter, and clothes. That luxury only appeared in my life when I turned 27, after spending five years in the national navy, chasing the dream of being the hero and the pride of my family.

But that dream was crushed not only by the corruption and lies of military life in a country where personal interests always outweigh social ones, but because I was miserable in a place where injustice, abuse, and cruelty were served hot, 24/7.

When I finally resigned from what had been my biggest dream, I came home empty-handed, no longer the family's pride. I felt like I had let down everyone who had admired me and sent me letters. I went from being the provider—the one who had extra money, who everyone talked about, who saw pride in his father's eyes—to a guy who played PlayStation eight hours a day, ate junk food, and would lie around doing nothing. I felt like I had wasted my life and that nothing would ever be the same.

Thankfully, my parents helped me find work. But the disappointment was brutal: after being one of the top students in my combat courses with some of the best physical test scores in the Navy, the only jobs I was offered were as a security guard or supervisor. That reality shattered what was left of my confidence, and I took the first job available—working with my father, who owned a window facade installation business. That job would lead to one of the biggest fights of my life: confronting the toxic relationship with my father and the mirror he held up to me.

One day, between work and playing soccer, my sister suggested I try a new sport: underwater rugby. I resisted at first, but eventually gave it a shot—and it became my escape from a boring, repetitive life. Playing a three-dimensional sport that forced me to be present with my body reignited a new love for life. It gave me reasons to work and save money to travel for tournaments.

For five years, everything felt good in the water. But on land, things kept getting worse. My relationship with my father deteriorated daily. Our fights were brutal. There was no respect left. The year my grandfather Fabio died, I decided to take a motorcycle trip to Bucaramanga, and I quit my job—no backup plan. After a heated argument, I just walked away from it all.

I have to admit, those were dark days. I tried everything, even webcam modeling. I sold empanadas outside training just to pay rent to my mom for my room.

One day, I decided to become a personal trainer. It started out of nowhere—through a post on a website—and it flowed naturally. Each month, I gained a new client. I remember telling myself, "If I make 1,500,000 pesos a month, I'll be happy," and just like that, it happened—no more, no less. I had enough to train, pay bills, and eat out.

But my restless mind wasn't satisfied. That inner spark led me to new people, new places—wealthier, healthier, more conscious folks. And I, a kid raised with strict basics, who had never known comfort or luxury, fell straight into that lifestyle.

I lost respect for my clients—I only cared about who paid more. I chased money, broke relationships, and abandoned the values and integrity that had defined me for years.

Eventually, I got tired of the same old thing—of people, routines, everything. Even the sport I once loved became joyless. I realized that nothing would ever be enough, because I was empty inside and trying to fill that hole with things from the outside.

After ten years in the sport, I had only one real friend. The rest either disliked or resented me—something I had cultivated myself through my ego, which wanted to crush others before being hurt again. I overheard things people said about me that really shocked me.

The space that once saved me became unbearable. I felt rejected by the world that once celebrated me. What used to be a dream became a nightmare. I clearly remember the day my body said, *Enough*.

It was during a tournament in my city. I was playing out of obligation, no longer excited or emotionally invested. During an ordinary match, I took a hit to the head that would've been no big deal any other day. But this time, it hurt like hell. For the first time, I felt real, soul-crushing pain. I left the game to check on myself and, while walking to our gear, about 15 meters from the pool, I collapsed, crying in front of 300 people who had once seen me as the strongest, coldest guy in the game. I couldn't stop. My body broke down in sobs. Even rival players came to check on me. And it was serious—at least to me.

I hadn't cried in years, let alone in public. That day, something inside me cracked. My armor couldn't take any more.

That marked the beginning of my second mental health crisis. Not only had I grown tired of the thing that made me money and gave me status, but my passion had become a source of pain. After three months of deep depression, I decided I wanted to end my life.

I said goodbye to my mom and some people close to me, and I went to a river in Buenaventura called La Serpentina. I asked nature to show me if there was a reason to live, and not only did it give me one, it gave me magic: a deep connection to the Earth and to my own essence. That trip changed my life and gave me reasons to continue healing through movement and knowledge.

It's been two years since that moment, and my quest for knowledge continues. Now I study how to heal the body through movement and emotions. It's still hard for me to explain what I do, but I'll try.

As a personal trainer, I learned the body is much more than a shell. True balance comes from moving your body, listening to your emotions, and feeding your mind. I began studying the body my own way, which led me to study the fascia—how it gets blocked by poor movement or toxic thoughts. I integrated that knowledge into my process, along with awareness of habits, and that's how I created what I call *healing in motion*. A method where I teach others (and myself) how to build a healthier, more conscious, more integrated relationship with the body and the self.

That same year, I wished to learn how to cry—and the world, the universe, in all its magic, brought me people, moments, and places so beautiful that I sometimes feel like a billionaire. And I'll admit—I still struggle to feel worthy of all the blessings life gives me. But peace is always a decision—a decision to be at peace with your heart, your soul, and your mind.

I won't lie—if you ask me what's been the hardest thing I've ever done in life, I'll tell you without a doubt: healing myself. Not surviving poverty, or the humiliation in the military, or the countless physical and mental challenges—no, none of that compares to the difficulty of healing emotionally. Of crying. Of being vulnerable. Of sharing myself honestly. Of accepting that I don't always have to be the strongest. Of realizing I was abused, and that it still hurts. Of begging for love and leaving myself last. Of wanting to belong, to fit in, to be seen. Of being afraid of humiliation, abandonment, and rejection.

It's a long road—sometimes lonely, painful, and hard. I've wanted to quit countless times. I've cried more this year than I have in my entire life. I've felt out of place, misunderstood, like maybe I'm wrong and should return to a life of distractions, pleasure, and numbing.

But even though it feels strange to live in peace, even though I'm still learning to talk to my shadows and fears, and even though my chest still aches for reasons I can't explain, I've seen love. The love that I am, the love I can give, and the love I can receive.

I've witnessed the power of being vulnerable, of helping others heal. The magic in my hands that guides people to a place where physical and emotional pain no longer exist. The gift of unconditional love I've been given—the ability to give without expecting anything back.

So, if you ask me for advice, I'll tell you: life is different for everyone. But if you came across my story, I want you to know that everything you've done matters. You should be proud of how far you've come, because only you know what you've had to go through to be where you are.

I love you.

ABOUT the AUTHOR

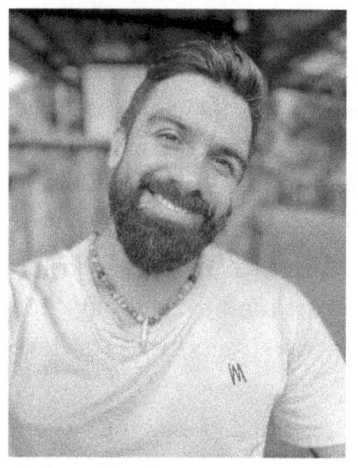

Juan Camilo Posada Arenas is a personal trainer, a movement healer, and a guide in fascia release techniques. For over seven years, he has dedicated his life to studying and supporting transformation through the body, understanding that movement is a gateway to emotional and spiritual healing. Before walking this path, he served five years in the Colombian Navy—an experience that shaped his character and taught him the true meaning of discipline and inner strength. At 36 years old, his greatest education has come from life itself—through scarcity, pain, and the relentless drive to keep moving forward. He has mastered multiple sports, studied health and anatomy deeply, and now channels all that energy into sharing what he's learned. His work is a bridge between body and soul. He works with those who seek to reconnect with themselves, reclaim their inner power, and heal—through movement—the places the mind alone cannot reach.

Social Link:
IG: @juanprimitiv

Chapter 6

You Are Not Alone

A Mental Health Nurse's Reflection on Men's Silent Battles

Christen E. Bryce, RN, MS

As a mental health nurse, I see people on the absolute worst days of their lives. Some wear their emotions on their sleeves, while others do whatever they can to convince us that they're "fine." Many will try to force a smile, strike up a "normal" conversation, and try to downplay the situation at hand to convince us to let them leave.

Even if they were brought to the hospital as a direct result of something they said or did that implied suicidality.

Even if they attempted to end their life.

I see the silent pain—the kind that you can't just ask someone to *rate on a scale from zero to ten*. The kind that won't show up on X-rays, tests, charts, or blood tests. And far too often, I see it in men. Men who appear to "have it all together," from the outside, but feel as though they are suffocating on the inside.

Society tells men to *be strong, take it like a man,* and expects them to hold the weight of the world on their shoulders without emoting. That's just how men should be, right? We want them to be kind, thoughtful, and nurturing—possibly even criticizing them for not being more sensitive, when it comes to romantic relationships and with their kids. But wait, don't be *too* emotional because *real men don't cry*.

From a very young age, boys are sent extremely mixed messages regarding emotions. They are taught to lead, but never falter. To "man up," push through, but never fall apart. We've created a culture where many men carry unbearable weight in silence. They don't always feel safe talking about their feelings, even to those who love them.

I'm not a man, and I'd never pretend to fully understand that experience. However, I am someone who's spent years in my professional life walking alongside people through their darkest days—listening, witnessing, and holding space. I've seen time and time again what happens when pain is left unspoken. In my personal life, I've been both a nurturer and provider for my own daughters. A mom who had to take on both parental roles when my oldest daughter's biological father opted to leave me when I was three months pregnant. I would never assert that a mother can *replace* a father's role. Actually, I can attest to the palpable void a family experiences without one. I'm also able to empathize with certain feelings that men have expressed, such as the fear, shame, worthlessness, disappointment in self, and embarrassment that comes along with not being sure if you can adequately provide for your family.

This chapter is for the men who fake being okay. For the ones who feel they can never catch up. For the dads trying to be everything to everyone, the partners who feel unseen, and the sons who grew up without room to cry or ask for a hug when they need one.

We need to talk about men's mental health, because it's costing lives. Statistically, males over 75 and between the ages of 25 and 44 are among the most likely to die by suicide. That's not a scare tactic. It's reality. Behind those numbers are real fathers, brothers, friends, husbands, sons. Some smiled in every photo. Some made us laugh. Some never once let on that they were struggling.

I knew one of them.

In 2016, while working in the ER crisis unit, I met one of my "phone friends" from the inpatient Mental Health Unit—a nurse who was sent to start cross-training with us. I'd only spoken to him over the phone regarding admissions until then. David was handsome, with a bright smile and sparkling eyes. His energy was intoxicating, warm, and comfortable. His sense of humor and wit were immediately apparent.

We quickly became "real" friends, and he even stopped by my new house to see how I was doing after my divorce was finalized, even though *he* had just had surgery. He brought Chinese food for lunch and played Candyland with my daughters and me. David was the kind of guy who was a classic gentleman and was everybody's buddy. He would walk us to our cars at night after our work shifts, to make sure we were safe. One of my favorite things about him was how highly he spoke of his beautiful wife. He absolutely adored her, their dogs, and going on adventures with them—he loved nature. There are so many things that made him unforgettable:

- He wore fun socks. It was his thing, and his socks always sparked conversations.
- He loved helping others and would have given anyone the shirt off his own back (which is probably why he'd often be stuck at work late charting).
- He saw nursing as part of his identity, after "husband" and "dog dad."
- He never complained about his hour-long commute.
- He would clock out, then wait for us to be finished so he could walk us out.
- He was hard on himself when learning new things, and this quality made him strive to be the best nurse that he could be –and boy, was he an amazing one!

To this day, David is one of the most thoughtful and compassionate people I've ever known, always carrying himself with humility, grace, and humor.

In September of 2017, we lost him.

When he was reported missing by his wife, one of the managers called me to see if I'd talked to him. I hadn't, so I immediately texted and called him to let him know that people were worried. I tried to believe the best. Maybe he just needed space. Maybe he went hiking to clear his head. But when his vehicle was found near a nature trail, we knew something was wrong.

A search party was organized, and we were split up into groups of about six or seven. The terrain was rough—brush, swamp, thick with vines. And even as we combed the area, my brain kept trying to convince me, "This isn't real." That we weren't actually looking for him, even when we came across a fairly fresh footprint about his size, then an empty Dunkin' Donuts coffee cup, followed by the lid to that cup. But it could have been from any hiker, right? It was just a coincidence. It *had* to be.

Not long before the end of our search shift, I had to leave. The rest of my group kept searching. After arriving home, my phone rang. My breath caught in my throat the second I saw the name of my friend who had still been there, but in another search group. I picked up, and the voice on the other end said the words I feared: *"We found his body."*

My legs gave out. I collapsed to the floor of my family room in sobs that made no sound. Silent grief. Paralyzed heartbreak. Once I could catch my breath and form a sentence, I asked her if she meant *her* group found him.

And then she told me, **"It was my search group that had found him."** I felt like a dagger shot through my chest. If my group found him, that meant it was David's own brother, his best friend, and the 18-year-old son of the friend on the other end of the phone.

I felt numb. I kept thinking, *God spared me from seeing that, but his poor brother and friend will have that scene forever etched in their memories.* I truly believe God protected me in that moment, because that would have broken me completely. Even now, I am thankful for that mercy.

The days that followed brought such a mix of emotions. In my mind, I couldn't stop picturing a made-up vision of his own brother and best friend finding him. I couldn't stop asking questions. How could someone so warm, so supportive, so empathetic, and especially a mental health professional who helps people who feel suicidal for a living, not reach out? How did he end up alone in that place? What did we miss?

We rehashed every memory. We asked ourselves if we should have noticed something, any red flags. We were mental health professionals, after all. We see depression every day.

But the truth is, the strongest smiles often hide the deepest pain.

That is how we missed it.

Because, as so many do, David knew how to hide it and what *not* to say. Once his pain was so deep, he knew exactly what to do and what not to do. I kept thinking about how he had just been at my house a few weeks earlier, playing a game with my kids, acting like his usual joyful self. Men are often so focused on carrying the weight of the world on their shoulders, but not "allowed" to emote properly while doing so, until it's too late for others to notice that *their* "cup" is empty.

That loss changed me. Forever.

Since then, I've become hyper-aware of the pain men carry in silence. I talk to them every day—men who feel overwhelmed, ashamed, exhausted, stuck. Men who are "doing everything right," and still feel like they're failing.

I've seen how society conditions men to swallow their emotions. I've heard the shame behind their words, even when they don't mean to say it out loud. And I've witnessed how loneliness piles on—quietly, relentlessly—until it becomes unbearable.

To every man reading this:

You are allowed to talk.

You are allowed to cry.

You are allowed to be unsure.

You are allowed to feel.

Being vulnerable is not a weakness. It is courage in its rawest form.

And to those who love them:

Check on your husbands.

Check on your brothers.

Check on your friends.

Let them know they don't have to be "fine" all the time.

Normalize honest conversations. Celebrate emotional strength. Make space for the pause, the breath, the "I don't know."

We've done an incredible job creating visibility for moms, for mental health, for resilience. Let's not leave men behind in the process.

Let's invite them in.

If this chapter makes you think of someone, text them. Call them. Hug them longer than usual.

That one moment of connection could be the lifeline they didn't know they needed.

You are not alone.

And neither are they.

ABOUT the AUTHOR

Christen is a board-certified psychiatric registered nurse, advocate, mentor, and author. She is also an Executive Contributor for Brainz Magazine. Christen works with a wide variety of clients struggling with mental health or relationship issues, with a primary focus on faith-based generational healing. Christen's mission is to empower adult children of late-life (grey) divorce and their families to take charge of their well-being before crises escalate in their own relationships. She is devoted to redefining mental wellness through Rational Emotive Behavioral Coaching and preventative care. As the founder of The Crisis Nurse, she developed The 6-Step CRISIS Plan to guide individuals in taking proactive steps toward emotional and psychological well-being. Through education, mentorship, and advocacy, Christen equips others with the tools to build resilience, embrace self-care, and cultivate a more fulfilling, sustainable life.

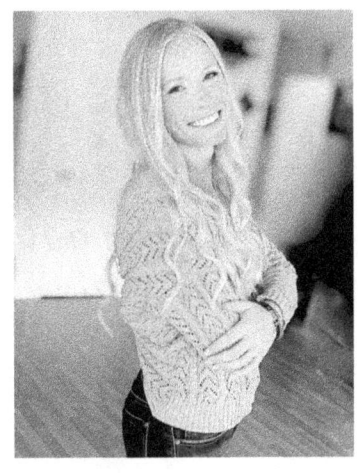

Her first solo book, *PIVOT: With My 6-Step Crisis Plan*, can currently be purchased, along with a companion journal.

Social Link:
linktr.ee/christenbryce_rn

Chapter 7

How To Be A Creative While Staying (Sorta) Sane

Federico Soto

Creativity. It's what made Homo habilis craft the first stone tool. It's the voice of the gods whispered directly into your mind in the form of epiphanies, fantasies, dreams. Without it, there's no wheel, no Renaissance, no Industrial Revolution, no Apollo 11 mission, no Sergeant Pepper, no Seinfeld, no sushi, and *definitively* no oral sex.

At a time when frightening technological advances can mimic many of what we used to consider human endeavors, true creativity has become the final stronghold for our species, and quite possibly, the most *uniquely human* trait you can tap into. And, at the nexus of creativity, lies that gooey center wherein emotions and ideas coalesce into awe-inspiring, thought-provoking, rebellion-inducing, sexy, sexy art.

But because the universe has a wicked sense of humor, the incredible superpower that is creativity is intrinsically linked to the shitshow that is your state of mind.

In plainer terms: whatever you're going through, mentally, is going to affect both the type of art you create and how productive you are at creating it. The thing is, there is no "one size fits all" answer to what your mental state *should be* when attempting a creative endeavor. To some people, being in a healthy, peaceful, mental state is the optimal for creation, whereas others won't even pick up the pen, paintbrush, camera, etc., if their whole life isn't on fire.

One thing is for sure though: the very traits that fuel creative expression (emotional sensitivity, deep introspection, heightened perception) can also make creative folk *more vulnerable* to mental health challenges. The gift of being able to experience emotions with greater intensity, notice subtleties that others overlook, and live with a rich inner world that feeds your work, comes with the drawback of also making you more susceptible to anxiety, depression, and a myriad of other psychological struggles, often exacerbated by the instability and pressures inherent with creative professions. It's like the medium who can talk to her dead relatives but is also prone to demonic possession, or put even more succinctly: there's no such thing as a "free lunch."

The good news is that *the creative process itself* can also be a powerful tool for managing and making sense of the mental health challenges you're more exposed to for being creative. Because the act of creating offers a way to *externalize* the inner chaos, to translate emotion into form, and to find meaning in pain. That's why many artists describe their work as "cathartic", because it provides them a way to process experiences that might otherwise feel overwhelming. Of course, this therapeutic quality of creativity doesn't negate the difficulty of the process, but it's the very thing that can provide relief, clarity, and even healing. Art is then both an outlet and a mirror, reflecting your internal state while offering a path forward. The only way out is through.

And that is the ugly truth behind creativity: maneuvering through the labyrinth that is your own mental terrain can be as important to your career as your artistic talent itself. Hell, maybe even more so, because what good is being a creative genius if your personal demons won't even let you finish that project? Thus, in this chapter I'm about to lay out all I know about the inextricable link between creative work and mental health, debunking some myths and sharing some tips I've learned along the way about this connection that isn't just some abstract concept, but the water we must swim in daily if we're thinking about making a career of this.

Quick disclaimer: I'm absolutely *not* a psychologist. I'm just a Colombian writer who stumbled into the creative industries about 20 years ago with a head full of stories and absolutely no idea how much the making of those stories would cost me mentally. My journey has taken me from publishing to film and back again, with oh-so-many detours in between. I've written for comics, children's books, movies, plays, video games, television, podcasts, and now this very chapter you're reading. Each new medium brought new challenges and fresh anxieties. Each project shadowed by the fear that it might be my last.

Because nobody prepares you for the crushing weight of deadline after deadline that just creeps up on you regardless of how many times you said you'd "get ahead of it this time"; the constantly comparing yourself to other artists knowing you'll never reach that level of mastery; and of course, the constant, paralyzing fear that someone will finally discover you're a fraud who has no business making art in the first place.

Sound familiar?

If it does, then this chapter is for you. And read on, because we're going to explore the question.

Why Do Creatives Mentally Struggle?

If you're a creative person, then odds are you're sensitive. And by "sensitive," I don't mean you're some kind of pathetic wimp, because it's 2025 and by now you should know that understanding, empathizing with, or even showing emotions doesn't make you any less of a man. Hemingway was sensitive and also tough as nails, so you can stop feeling insecure about being in tune with emotions because that's where creativity comes from.

However, like I mentioned before, it's that same sensitivity that fuels your work, which *also* makes you more vulnerable to psychological strain. Add to that the difficult external conditions that often accompany creative work (unstable income, constant rejection, intense competition, and public scrutiny), and you get the ideal conditions for issues like burnout, impostor syndrome, anxiety, depression, or even substance abuse. All of which I unfortunately know quite well, so let me blast through these in case you're going through some of these too.

Burnout is *more* than just fatigue. It's the erosion of work you *used* to take joy in doing, a loss of connection to the creative projects that once gave you purpose, and it feels like having your brain pummeled into jelly while also running a marathon. It fucking sucks and I should know, because I've not only experienced it firsthand, I've also seen it happen quite often. Back when I tried to run a production company, I was wearing every hat possible: creating, editing, and producing nonstop until my once interminable well of creativity ran dry. As an editor, I watched young creators push through impossible deadlines, telling themselves they'd rest after just one more project, but there was *always* another project hot on the heels of the previous one, and they needed money to make ends meet so they always ended up taking it and pushing back that rest period just a little more. Many eventually burned out completely and wound up abandoning the work they once loved doing.

Impostor syndrome is an issue I've seen envelop artists of all disciplines and backgrounds, regardless of their levels of experience, commitment, or success. It's that nagging, unignorable inner voice whispering that your success was a fluke and that you don't belong in the same conversation as other *real* artists around you. I've seen best-selling authors, popular actors, and award-winning musicians totally crumble under the weight of their own inner critics. Oftentimes, the more you've achieved as an artist, the louder that voice gets because there is now greater pressure to maintain the success you've had. Thus, the fear that you'll eventually be exposed as a fraud becomes overwhelming, and you end up creatively paralyzed, ironically proving the voices right.

Anxiety and perfectionism mostly come together, like a yummy broken glass and barbed wire sandwich. Perfectionism is typically *the result of* the anxiety you feel about having your editor, director, or audience like your art. So, you obsess over every little detail and second-guess every choice because you're striving for the unreachable. And to make matters worse, nowadays, you have things like social media that amplify this feeling by turning each creative act into a public performance where feedback is immediate and often harsh. (Have you *seen* that YouTube comment section? It's the worst place ever.) I've seen creatives get into the habit of redoing their work dozens of times, not because it wasn't good, but because it wasn't *perfect*, and the result was always the same: missed deadlines and stalled projects.

There are only two things that seem to be *everywhere* these days: Pedro Pascal and depression. Since the latter is slightly more ubiquitous (for now), I won't spend that much time explaining what depression is, but rather illustrate how this condition introduces a different set of challenges for creative folk. No shade on the people who have jobs that don't demand them to be creative (God knows I envy them so much sometimes), but the fact is that it's probably easier to drive a forklift when depressed than it is to make art when you're depressed. Notice how I said easier and not easy because *nothing* comes easy when depressed. However, when that "black dog" strikes a creative person, it silences the inner voice that once wanted them to create. They feel utterly disconnected from that force that allowed them to have almost supernatural abilities, and like Obi-Wan Kenobi in that mediocre Disney+ show, they go from Jedi knight to old man with a glow stick faster than you can say, "Come on, that show wasn't that bad, Darth Vader was sick in that." Depression makes the stories that once felt urgent suddenly feel meaningless, and unfortunately, this is when most of us turn to substances for solace.

For some, substance use becomes a method of coping, but the brief respite that a substance can temporarily give you is a slippery slope towards abuse and addiction. Again, I (regretfully) have some personal insight on the matter. I started using substances near the start of my career, back when I was working as a unit director for a taping of the X-Factor…yeah, that show that's like 90% people embarrassing themselves during the audition process and then 10% actual musical game show. The call times were hellish. It was my first time working on something of that magnitude, and I was just starting a very meaningful relationship; it was just a lot to juggle at the time. So, I started using, just to relax, just enough to get some sleep, just to have a mini-vacation amongst an onslaught of challenging work. Well, the X-Factor came and went, so did the next project, and even that special relationship I mentioned, but you know what solace I had? The drugs.

The image of the addicted genius is dangerously romanticized, even I fell for it for a time, thinking, *hell, if Jordan Peele, The Beatles, Seth Rogen, Bill Maher, and practically every rapper out there can do amazing art while on drugs, I can probably get baked and write this script, no?"* No. While *some* creatives can create while under the influence, substances don't really enhance creativity in any significant way. Drugs aren't like steroids for bodybuilders, other than when they fuck up their lives in the long run, and now, they need to take *other* stuff to get a boner. Also (and trust me on this), you are *not* Jordan Peele, The Beatles, Seth Rogen, Bill Maher, or Lil' Wayne. They can write *"Get Out"* while totally baked; you will just get Taco Bell and pass out on your couch watching cartoons. They are the exception; you are the rule. For every hyper-successful drug user, there are a million more whose drug use actually *hindered* their progress, and not to get all Nancy Reagan on you, but you probably want to run those numbers *before* you decide to make substances your crutch for creativity.

If you're like me, you probably thought you needed those substances to be like the artists you idolized, but keep in mind creativity thrives on presence, not oblivion; and that idea that you need to be like a sort of person to produce a type of art is not only toxic but also dead wrong.

In fact, let's take a look at the validity of the old.

Myth of the Crazed Artist

Our culture idolizes the vision of the tortured artist who is mentally unwell. It's the notion that suffering (physical or mental) is the inevitable toll for achieving artistic brilliance. It's the belief that mental anguish is not only pervasive among creators but somehow makes their work *more* authentic. Noble, even necessary. It's easy to buy into this myth because the stereotype is everywhere, creating a mystique around madness, suggesting that the creative mind must first be broken in order to then be brilliant. Look, Van Gogh didn't cut his ear off because he was so well-adjusted, and it's not like we ever got to see what Kurt Cobain's "greatest hits" era would've looked like, so there *must* be something to it, right?

Wrong. This narrative is *poison*. A falsehood. A toxic fable that glorifies agony and overlooks the destruction mental health issues can leave in their wake. Trust me, there is nothing glamorous about anxiety so crippling that you miss deadlines; nothing inspiring about alienating collaborators, friends, and family during a manic episode; and I don't care how cool that new song is, there isn't any heroism in having your life fall apart because of depression.

This myth takes real victims. Causes genuine suffering. It tells us that if we're not in the throes of unbearable pain, our work must be trivial or shallow. That if we dare seek help to manage our mental state, then we're dulling the sharp edge that makes our art cut deep. But the truth is that creativity doesn't really prosper in chaos; it *needs* clarity like a seed needs water and sunshine to flourish. Sure, you may *have had that idea* back when you were a mess, but you need some semblance of mental normalcy so as to execute it to its full potential. Like Hemingway said, "Write drunk, edit sober."

There's this idea that only a certain type of person can produce a specific kind of thing. But you don't have to be a tortured soul to make people cry with your melancholic works of art, just like you don't have to be Captain Sunshine to make upbeat, feel-good creations. It's the whole reason why super approachable, happy-go-lucky manga artist Junji Ito can make macabre horror stories that make you shit your pants like "Uzumaki" and "Smashed", while a demanding, unempathetic despot like Hideo Miyazaki can produce emotionally touching movies like "Ponyo," "My Neighbor Totoro," or "Princess Mononoke."

Remember: creative people are nuanced human beings who have bad days and go through changes just like everyone else. So don't try to fit into some harmful mold, thinking you have to be this way to create this kind of art. Just produce whatever is inside you at any given time. If Tupac wrote both "Dear Mama" and "Hit 'em up," then you, too, are allowed to create all over the emotional, moral, or philosophical spectrum without being judged or labeled for it.

The key takeaway is that we don't have to be in X or Y mental state to produce X or Y kind of art, but rather that we need to learn how to work with our own mind, however it is. When we give ourselves the chance to develop emotional literacy and sustainable practices, our work not only becomes more consistent but also more *profound* than we ever thought possible. Acknowledging that the creative mind needs care makes space for both our art and our mental health to coexist, and even enrich one another. In the end, it's not a choice between sanity and success, but the challenge to integrate the two, to understand that mental health and creativity influence each other, and to develop strategies that allow creators to nurture both.

What are some of those strategies? Glad you asked.

The Ol' Mental Wellness Toolbox

While it's true that you don't need to be in perfect mental health in order to produce a creative project, there are some healthy strategies that you can use if you want to nudge your mind into a more creative-friendly space. I've seen these tools work in both myself and the many artists I've worked with. Here's hoping they can help you, too.

Stay Creative in the Chaos

Look, you're not always going to be in the mood for making art. Still, what truly differentiates the hobbyist from the professional is the ability to just grit your teeth and get the work done, no matter how you feel or what may be going on with your life externally. Some deadlines are written in stone, with the blood of all those who weren't able to meet them, and in those cases, it pays to know how to put your brain in "creative mode."

The way I see it, there are two main strategies you can implement when having to create through the fog that clouds your mind. The first one is quite simple and probably more appealing to you "stoic" types reading this: *Just sit your ass down and do the work.* Yeah, I know it seems like the most idiotic answer ever, but have you heard of "Occam's Razor"? It's a principle asserting that the simplest explanation is usually the best one. Well, this is that. Plus, it's been proven that just starting a creative project and working on it (even if the output is shit at first) eventually kicks your brain into the creative gear, like starting a car by pushing it. If you're not convinced yet, legendary Spanish artist Pablo Picasso pointed at this very practice when he said, "Let the muse catch you at work." And who are we to doubt Picasso? People use his name as shorthand for when somebody paints well, for fucks sake!

Now, if the first tip was for the simple, relentless stoics, then the next tip is a little more for you, Jungian pop-psychologists. It's called "compassionate compartmentalizing" and it's a stress management technique that helps you separate aspects of your life or emotions into "compartments" where you still allow yourself to process them when you're ready while also giving yourself the space you need to complete that urgent task without crying hysterically or making an ass out of yourself at the office Christmas party.

In "compassionate compartmentalizing," you acknowledge your pain, then give yourself permission to set it aside *temporarily* and do the work. This technique is all about separating your *identity* from your *output*. One bad page doesn't mean you're a bad writer. Even Michael Jordan had some off nights, so don't be so hard on yourself! As a matter of fact, give your inner critic a name. (I call mine "Jose" after a friend who is literally the biggest hater on planet earth.) Ask the critic to step aside until it's time to revise. Then go to your workstation and just *play*. Doodle, write something silly, break the pressure of perfection, but just *get busy*. Soon enough, you'll see you're back at work without even noticing.

Turn Her into Literature

Henry Miller said, "The best way to get over a woman is to turn her into literature." What Miller was talking about was the idea that your pain can become creative material, but it needs transformation. After reading the first part of this chapter, you know you don't have to suffer to be an artist, but when messed-up shit *does* happen to you, don't just vent, *craft*. Take your negative, low-vibrational feelings and use some emotional alchemy to turn them into something productive. It's the whole idea behind the psychological concept of *sublimation*.

In sublimation, your brain takes those spicy, primal urges you may feel during stressful times (like aggression, horniness, and aggressive horniness) and, rather than falling into some ethically or morally reprehensible activities, chooses to do something *constructive* with that energy instead. So now you're doing ballet instead of holding up a liquor store. You're channeling your inner chaos into something society gives you a fist bump for instead of a restraining order.

Know When to Hold 'em, Know When to Fold 'em.

Yes, I just quoted a Kenny Rogers song, but before you throw this book into a fiery pit, know this: there are times when pushing through isn't brave—it's harmful. And if you've ever been in a writer's room that goes on all night, you know that there's a point of diminishing returns for your creative work. If you're not careful about identifying that point, you may just replace an idea that had artistic value with some dribble you spat out at 11:45 pm when your brain was on airplane mode.

Know the warning signs of burnout, my friends! Irritability, disinterest, fantasizing about pummeling your client until there's blood in their stool, physical symptoms, etc. Be aware when your own body is telling you to chill and take a step back before you collapse. Taking some time to rest and go back at it later isn't laziness, it's *strategy*. You can stay connected to creativity through journaling, reading, idea sketching, or any sort of "lighter" creative process if you want to take it down a notch, but if you want to shut that part of your brain down for the night and come back stronger at a later date, that's cool too.

Just be sure to *rest*.

Maintain Good Habits. (Duh.)

By now, we've covered that creativity needs a clear, healthy mind to do its thing. Well, that starts with the basics: get some sleep. Not the half-awake kind where you're scrolling in bed, but the real, drool-on-the-pillow kind. Your brain runs the whole show, so give it what it needs to function.

Moving your body helps, too. Nothing fancy, a walk, a stretch, even doing some pushups in the kitchen in between calls, can make a big difference. Physical movement gets the mental gears turning, and it's one of the quickest ways to reset when you're feeling stuck.

This is kind of a no-brainer, but it also helps to cut down on all the digital noise. Notifications, emails, and endless scrolling might feel like background noise, but they take up more mental space than you realize. Try setting some boundaries around screen time, especially when you're trying to create. Simple rituals like lighting a candle before you begin or closing a notebook when you're done can trick your mind into powering down. These little signals tell your brain it's time to shift gears, and over time, they help carve out a mental space that's just for your work.

Most importantly, learn to notice your own rhythms without getting all judgy about them. Some days the ideas flow clearly like a crystalline river; other days they're murkier than Michigan tap water (apologies to the good people of Flint, Michigan). That's normal; the ebbs and flows are what make the work rich, but they can also wear you out if you don't take care of yourself. Remember: protecting your mental space isn't some bogus self-care trend. It's how you make sure there's room for your best ideas to grow.

Wholeness > Hustle

I'm gonna level with you: taking care of myself hasn't dulled my creativity; it's actually what's kept it alive. I've learned that sustainable creativity isn't about hitting a word count or making something brilliant every Tuesday. It's about weaving your creative life *into* the rest of your life, like a slightly less depressing version of the AIDS Memorial Quilt. I'm a writer on the days I write *and* on the days I stare at my ceiling, wondering if liking cheese counts as a personality. My creative identity isn't hanging by a thread every time I have a slow week. It's now *built into me*, baked into the way I see and feel and process the world, whether or not I've made anything lately.

And hey, you don't have to do this alone. Find your people, the ones who get that some days you're a genius and other days, you forget how to spell "genius." Be clear about what you need—whether it's feedback, encouragement, or someone to tell you to close the 19 tabs in your browser. Get help when things get heavy. Be honest with your collaborators. Most folks don't need you to be perfect; they'll settle for *real*. Do I still get nervous staring down a blank page? Yes. Do I still hear José, the inner critic, yammering away like he's auditioning for the shittiest one-man show? You betcha. The difference is now I've learned to make room for *all of it*. Because this whole creative thing isn't about control; it's about a relationship. Some days it's a love story, some days it's a sitcom, occasionally it's a porno, but more often than not, it's a horror movie. Whatever way it manifests for you on a given day, just remember that what truly matters is how you show up for it: messy, honest, and (hopefully) fully yourself.

ABOUT the AUTHOR

Federico Soto is a Colombian writer who specializes in storytelling and IP development. He's published two children's books (with one more on the way), a graphic novel, an indie comic book, and he has written or consulted for more than a dozen audiovisual projects in both the U.S. and Colombia. As an editor, he's worked for the popular Korean webcomic company *WebToon*, Florida-based LGBTQ+ magazine *Watermark Publishing*, and currently, for Indian podcasting/webcomic behemoth: *PocketFM*.

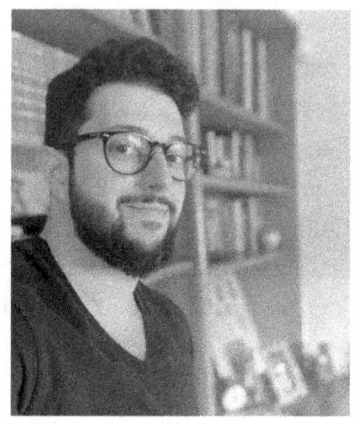

Safe to say Federico has worn many hats, even though he really *hates* wearing hats 'cause he can't pull 'em off (it's his face, it's weird). Maybe a fedora, though, on Halloween, if he's cosplaying Indiana Jones or something.

Social Links:
   IG @fedsoto
   X @KikoSoto

Chapter 8

Mission Accepted

Become the Man You Admire
Alan James Duro

I was in my early 30s, sitting alone in my apartment on a February night in Boston.

It was cold, dark, and I was right in the middle of a classic Nor'easter snowstorm. I lived with my girlfriend, but we were in the process of breaking up. She went to stay at her parents' house for the weekend. In addition to the breakup, I had been recently let go from my job, and I was collecting unemployment.

I had an idea in mind for a business, but I had no clients. Anxiety, fear, and sadness began to consume me. This wasn't the path I was meant to be on. I felt weak. I felt unconfident. I felt unsure of my next move. In short, I felt like a failure.

As I sat in silence on the couch, I couldn't help but ask: *Who am I becoming?*

I didn't have a clear answer.

As I sat there in despair, I did what most millennials did in the mid-2010s in moments like these: I went on YouTube. As I browsed aimlessly, my algorithm served up a random video about *"inversion thinking,* which was made famous by the late great investor Charlie Munger. The video explained that inversion thinking involves solving problems by looking at them from the reverse perspective. So I decided to give it a shot.

Instead of asking *Who am I becoming?* I inverted the problem and asked, *Who am I NOT becoming?* I thought long and hard about my life and all the men I've looked up to over the years since I was a kid. As I continued to think, the funniest person kept popping up in my mind. It was Bond... James Bond.

That's right. The "shaken-not-stirred" guy from the movies. Sean Connery, Daniel Craig, Roger Moore: take your pick. James Bond stood out to me as the polar opposite of how I felt. He's cool under pressure, physically capable, stylish, sophisticated, and totally in control. I felt like a lot of things at that moment, but one person that I certainly **did NOT** feel like was James Bond.

And that contrast gave me a strange kind of clarity. If I didn't know exactly who I wanted to become, at least I knew somebody whom I wanted to be *more like*. And for me, that became a starting point.

"If you can't figure out where to go, figure out who to be."

— Alan "James" Duro

The Importance of Role Models

I believe we all need something or someone to aim at. Some men have strong mentors, others have coaches or older brothers. I grew up with British parents and a stack of VHS James Bond movies that my Dad collected.

As a kid, I didn't understand half of what was going on in the films, but I knew one thing for sure: this guy James Bond was *the man*. The movies had action, adventure, and beating up bad guys; all things that appealed to a young boy. Also, when I watched the movies, I was always watching them with my Dad. I looked up to my Dad, and I knew that he also thought Bond was cool. So naturally, I wanted to be more like him, too.

As I got older and got serious about personal development, I realized that life isn't about reinventing the wheel. Most things you want to be or do have already been done—and there are people out there, both real and fictional, who've left blueprints.

You can just pick one and follow it.

When I looked at my scattered goals for my life: become financially free, build confidence, get in shape, improve relationships, travel the world, stay calm under pressure, etc. I realized I wasn't looking for a list. I was looking for an *identity* to step into. And that identity, for me, looked a lot like James Bond.

"If you want to be successful, find someone who has achieved the results you want and copy what they do."

— Tony Robbins

Why James Bond?

Let's break it down. Bond isn't just some playboy with gadgets. He's a master archetype. Especially for men trying to reclaim their sense of direction and purpose. Here's why:

- **He's in shape, but not a meathead.** He's athletic, mobile, strong, but never bulky or overdone. He trains for function, not vanity, and is extremely physically capable.
- **He's highly competent.** He can drive anything, fly anything, scuba dive, ski, shoot, and fight. He's basically a walking Swiss army knife. There's seemingly nothing he doesn't know how to do.
- **He can defend himself (and others).** He's not looking for a fight, but he's able to use violence if necessary. He moves

with the quiet confidence of a man who knows he'll be okay in any situation.
- **He's got incredible style.** James has a timeless quality. He always looks sharp and dressed appropriately for the occasion.
- **He's seemingly unbothered by money.** You never hear Bond talking about money, but he's clearly unencumbered by it. You never see him checking his bank balance or stressing about paying a parking ticket. He's free essentially, and *that's* the real dream.
- **He's well-traveled, cultured, and adaptable.** Whether he's in a market in Istanbul, having cocktails in Havana, or getting a suit tailored in London, he's comfortable anywhere. He knows the wine to order and the language to order it in. A true international man of mystery.
- **He attracts women. And not because he tries, but because of who he is.** He always gets the girl, but he's never chasing her. He's never needy or possessive. His mission comes first, and women are drawn to that.
- **He has a mission.** This is the key. Bond's not aimlessly wandering. Everything he does serves a greater purpose, and it's always a force for the greater good. His mission objective is the driver of almost everything he does, and that's what makes him so magnetic.

Becoming Bond: My Real-Life Mission

When I started to take this idea seriously, I asked myself: *What would it actually take to become more like James Bond?* Not as a fantasy, but as a guiding identity that I could align myself with in real life.

So I reverse-engineered it.

- What skills would I need to build?
- What habits?
- What kind of mindset?

Here's where I started:

- **Entrepreneurship & Financial Freedom:** I read books, took courses, and learned how to invest. Mastered sales, negotiation, and communication. Over time, I got my business off the ground and started investing in real estate.
- **Self-Defense & Confidence:** I started training in Jiu-Jitsu and Muay Thai. I got serious about consistent workouts to build strength, mobility, and discipline.
- **Calmness of Mind:** I read books on Stoic philosophy. I learned to meditate, developed emotional control, and started a journaling practice.
- **Appearance:** I invested in timeless wardrobe pieces that fit well and leaned into my personal style. Learned grooming habits that fit my lifestyle.
- **Worldliness:** After getting my online business going, I traveled. A TON. I learned Spanish. Immersed myself in new cultures. Practiced becoming comfortable in unfamiliar environments.

Bit by bit, I started to feel like a man who was *becoming something*. Not perfect, not Bond, but better than the guy who felt so lost and aimless that night in that apartment in Boston.

"Success is nothing more than a few simple disciplines, practiced every day."

— Jim Rohn

Create Your Own Archetype

Here's the thing: your "Bond" might not be James Bond. Maybe it's Muhammad Ali. Maybe it's Maximus from *Gladiator*. Maybe it's your grandfather.

The point isn't to copy someone else's life. The point is to use an archetype as a compass—something to aim at when you don't know where to go or what direction to take.

Ask yourself:

- *Who did I admire as a kid? Why?*
- *Who are the men I admire now? What traits do they embody?*
- *What kind of man would I be proud to become?*

When things get hard, when you feel lost, and when motivation runs dry, that archetype becomes your North Star. And when you're unsure what to do next, ask: *What would he do?*

It's not about pretending to be someone else. It's about becoming the man you were meant to be all along.

Final Thought

James Bond's character might be fictional, but that night in Boston, he gave me something real: direction. I wasn't lost. I just needed a version of myself I could believe in again.

So next time you're feeling lost, don't wait to feel ready. Pick your archetype. Study him. Train. Improve. Refine.

Make decisions today that your future self will thank you for.

You're not here to drift. You're here to *become*.

Make your time on this planet count.

Your mission starts now.

Additional Resources:

Chat GPT Prompts:

Potential prompts to put into ChatGPT to help you in your journey to finding a role model or archetype to follow.

1. **Identify Your Archetype**

- "*I feel lost and lack direction in my life. Help me identify a male role model or archetype that aligns with my values and the type of person I aspire to become. Provide three potential archetypes, explain their defining traits, and suggest specific habits or actions I can adopt to embody each one.*"

2. **Create Your Bond Blueprint**
    - "*I want to become a more confident, capable, and well-rounded man like James Bond. Break down the key traits and skills that define Bond and help me create a practical, actionable plan to develop each trait over the next 90 days. Include recommended books, exercises, and daily habits.*"

3. **Find Your North Star**
    - "*I struggle with motivation and feel stuck in a rut. Help me define a personal 'North Star' using a fictional character, historical figure, or real-life role model. Identify the qualities that make them compelling, outline how I can adopt similar traits, and provide three daily practices to stay aligned with this new identity.*"

For a comprehensive list of James Bond skills, a style guide, and a travel list to follow, scan the QR below and you'll receive free access to these resources.

ABOUT the AUTHOR

Alan James Duro is a Boston-born entrepreneur and real estate investor with deep ties to Nantucket Island in Massachusetts. His current home base is Medellín, Colombia, where he lives out part of his mission to create a life of freedom, adventure, and philanthropy through remote wealth building. He's the founder of **NextWave**, a company that helps clients in the senior care industry improve their sales operations. He's also a partner in **Stowe Holdings**, investing alongside his brother in multifamily real estate projects across the United States. Alan splits his time between scaling businesses, martial arts training, playing tennis, and exploring the world. An international man of mystery in training.

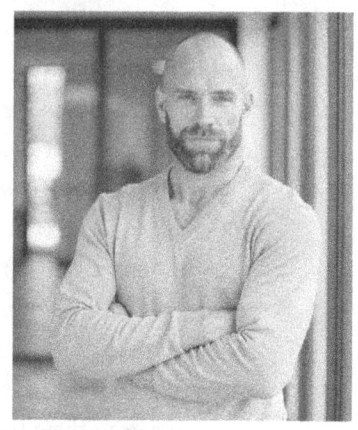

Social Link:
linktr.ee/alanjamesduro

Chapter 9

Breaking the Code

Redefining Self-Worth, Masculinity, and Success

Roje Khalique

Introduction

As a therapist, I have been privileged to be entrusted with truths that rarely get voiced out loud. I witness how in all individuals, self-worth is either nurtured or quietly eroded over time. I hear the pain behind conversations about masculinity, how it's being dismantled in public discourse, often without offering a healthy or grounded alternative. I also see how society equates success with money, power, and status, frequently at the cost of relationships, emotional well-being, and collective harmony.

The insights I share in this chapter are drawn from years of clinical work with a great many men facing depression, anxiety, and low self-esteem. These reflections stem from the therapeutic space, and whilst they are meaningful, they are not representative of all men. As a female therapist, I also acknowledge the limitations of my perspective.

This chapter is not intended to provide an exhaustive analysis across all ages, cultures, socioeconomic backgrounds, or gender identities, recognising that these patterns may manifest differently across racial, ethnic, and economic contexts where men face additional cultural expectations or systemic pressures. Nor does it aim to fully capture the complexity of mental health conditions such as depression, anxiety, and low self-esteem. Rather, it aims to shed light on recurring patterns I have encountered, patterns that warrant deeper attention in both public dialogue and professional spaces, including schools and home.

> "I didn't need my dad to be rich. I needed him to be reliable and emotionally available."

This statement, spoken by a successful CEO in my therapy room, captures a painful truth I've witnessed repeatedly across years of clinical practice: many men suffer in silence. Beneath layers of resilience, humour, or anger lies an unspoken story, often rooted in boyhood, that remains unresolved. I have sat with CEOs, fathers, and young professionals alike, each carrying the weight of unexpressed grief, confusion about their purpose, profound emotional exhaustion, and suppression.

Many boys (and girls) face intense pressure to meet academic standards and be at the top of their class, which shapes their early perception of self-worth. Second, boys often experience confusion about what it truly means to be a man in today's world. Third, there is overwhelming pressure to define their worth solely through material success.

Ultimately, the profound fear of judgment, fear of failure, and fear of rejection if they do not meet these societal expectations from a young age, reinforced throughout adolescence and manhood, often manifests as the pervasive anxiety of not measuring up and the dread of inadequacy, adding to their struggles with their mental and emotional health.

1. The Impact of Early Programming: Low Self-esteem and Childhood Conditioning

The boy who wasn't allowed to cry or share his pain grows into the man

who hides his distress, often for years, behind a mask that society accepts, but his heart does not.

This pattern often begins in childhood, where a boy may internalise the belief: *My worth is in making my parents happy, I must always achieve, I must never show weakness, I must never fail,* or *they'll think I'm not good enough.*

Over time, this mindset can create a deep-seated fear of judgment and failure. Boys who grow up with this pressure may channel it into external achievements, which can manifest as behavioural issues or academic stress in childhood. As they mature, some boys carry these same patterns into adulthood, where they may experience career burnout, emotional disconnection, or difficulties in relationships.

For many, their sense of self becomes closely tied to meeting expectations, whether set by parents, teachers, or peers, leading to a persistent fear of disapproval. As they move into adulthood, these pressures often intensify, as does the internalized ultimate fear of judgment and failure.

These clinical patterns align with research by Gerdes et al. (2021), who describes the "boy code" as a cultural script that teaches boys to suppress vulnerability and display strength, often at the expense of emotional and mental well-being. The fear of failure deepens when achievement is equated with worthiness from an early age.

The Cycle of External Validation

This pressure to achieve can lead to an unhealthy level of perfectionism, often revealing itself in a cycle between anxiety and depression. Anxiety is driven by a fear of failing (*I must not fail*) while depression sets in when the individual feels they've already failed; *I've let everyone down.* Consequently, they oscillate between these emotional states because, deep down, their self-worth has become tied to achievement.

This underlying belief, *I am only worthy if I succeed,* fuels the cycle. To escape these feelings, many turn to external validation, becoming hyper-focused on academic success, athletic dominance, physical perfection, romantic pursuits, or professional accolades. All the while, the emotional toll remains hidden beneath the surface.

Developing Internal Worth

Self-worth must be cultivated from the inside out, beginning in early childhood. When love and approval are conditional, tied solely to academic achievement, this can create an internal script that undermines emotional and mental well-being. I often hear men say things like, *Dad only wanted to show me off,* or *I was only good enough if I passed my exams.* High achievers are sometimes driven by an unconscious need to prove themselves, which can manifest as unhealthy perfectionism (*I need to be perfect, or I'm worthless*) or persistent impostor syndrome (*They'll find out that I'm not good enough.*) These patterns frequently come at the expense of emotional, mental, and even physical health.

Parents, teachers, and mentors play a critical role in helping boys uncover their intrinsic value. While academic and professional success are important, so too are emotional literacy, meaningful relationships, teamwork, creativity, life skills, and a sense of contribution to others. Carol Dweck's 2006 research on the growth mindset reinforces this belief that abilities can be developed, not fixed. When boys are encouraged to value effort, not just outcomes, they learn not to fear failure, and they tend to show greater psychological flexibility and well-being.

It's crucial for boys to learn from a young age that effort, overcoming challenges, and building resilience from failure (not being at the top or not passing) are just as important as test scores or future earnings. Yet many grow up internalising the message that their worth is defined solely by performance, be it academic grades, athletic wins, or future financial success. The result? A generation of boys chasing ever-shifting goalposts, often feeling like they're falling short no matter how hard they try.

These dynamics can be further complicated by cultural background. Men from different ethnic communities often navigate additional layers of expectation: the pressure to be the sole family provider, stereotypes based on race, or the tension between traditional cultural values and contemporary Western ideals of masculinity, can all add to the mental and emotional load.

Building Resilience: Celebrating Effort Over Perfection

We must celebrate effort and on-going personal growth. Consider, for example, telling a child, "*You can't spell,*" without recognising their genuine efforts reinforces the belief that only perfection earns praise. In therapy, many men trace their inner critic back to these early childhood moments, when well-meaning adults inadvertently equated mistakes with inadequacy. Over time, this message may be echoed by peers, managers, and loved ones.

By creating emotionally intelligent environments, where boys are seen, heard, and encouraged, we can raise a generation of men who feel worthy not because they have 'earned it', but because they have 'owned it' from the start.

A longitudinal study by Kiselica and Englar-Carlson (2010) supports these approaches, showing that targeted emotional development programs for boys significantly improve self-esteem and emotional literacy. It is essential that boys are provided with safe spaces to openly express their feelings without fear of judgment or stigma, helping to break the cycle of seeing failure as a sign of worthlessness. Research highlights that resilience is strengthened through experiencing and learning from failure, showing that setbacks are a normal and important part of personal growth (Carlson, 2024). In fact, through therapy, it becomes clear that for some men (and women), the pursuit of perfection may sustain the fear of failure.

Recommendations for Building Healthy Self-Worth in Boys

1. **Introduce mental health education** in schools to support boys' emotional development and self-worth.

2. **Train educators** to identify perfectionism and fear of failure, using strategies that emphasise effort, growth, and resilience.
3. **Shift praise** from achievement-focused to valuing effort and commitment, and supporting parents to reflect on how their praise shapes their sons' self-esteem and identity.
4. **Create safe spaces** where boys can express vulnerability, normalising it as a strength rather than a weakness.

2. Letting Men Define Masculinity: The Rigidity of Identity

Just as women rightly reject being defined by men, men deserve the same respect to explore and express their identities on their own terms.

Many men struggling with their mental health report a deep identity crisis, shaped by uncertainty around what it means to be masculine today. Amid shifting societal expectations, they often feel unable to express themselves without fear of judgment or shame. One core issue is that masculinity is increasingly being defined for men, often by others, including public discourse that has often been led by women.

Research by Levant and Richmond (2016) highlights how rigid gender role expectations can result in 'gender role conflict', which significantly correlates with depression and anxiety. It's not gender itself that causes harm, but the rigid, narrow definitions of how one 'should' be a man that often creates psychological distress.

Misuse of Clinical Labels and Misunderstanding of Masculinity

A concerning trend has emerged in the casual use of clinical terms like *'toxic masculinity'* and *'narcissism'*, especially on social media and popular wellness psychology. An increasing number of women describe previous male partners or relatives with these labels without fully understanding their clinical significance. Frequently, what appears as diagnosable disorders can in fact be relational breakdowns, unmet emotional needs, or simple miscommunication.

This is not to dismiss women's experiences or the reality of abuse. Rather, it calls for a clear distinction between emotional incompatibility and genuine psychological harm. Overusing clinical language dilutes the seriousness of real trauma and abuse and contributes to the blanket vilification of men and masculinity.

Originally, *'toxic masculinity'* was meant to critique harmful behaviours, and whilst some find this framework helpful for self-reflection, it is often misapplied in ways that shame all expressions of masculinity. Most men are not abusers or emotionally unavailable. Yet many feel blamed, misunderstood, or silenced, though some therapeutic approaches might emphasise different aspects of these dynamics. Some clients are labelled "*emotionally abusive*" or "*narcissistic*" not due to actual abuse or violence but because of emotional struggle, poor communication, or difficulty setting boundaries. These are serious clinical labels that must be used responsibly. Misusing them undermines their meaning and harms everyone involved.

Furthermore, If men are told that instincts like protectiveness, leadership, and provision are problematic, they may suppress healthy aspects of themselves. Protectiveness does not equal control, provision does not equal ego, and leadership does not equal dominance. When boys grow up hearing that masculinity is inherently dangerous or shameful, they may internalise the belief that something is wrong with their identity simply for 'being male'.

Without evolution in how schools, families, and mental health services approach masculinity, we risk raising boys who feel ashamed of their identity and are unsure of their role in society. Being a man should not mean suppression, guilt, or blame. Like girls, boys deserve affirmation. When traditional male roles such as providing, protecting, and leading are devalued or distorted, boys can become confused, and men can feel adrift.

Conflicting Expectations of Masculinity

Men today are caught between contradictory messages. Historically, men were socialised and encouraged to be stoic and emotionally restrained; now, society often criticises men for being "emotionally unavailable." Whilst feminism has rightly challenged outdated gender roles and empowered women, there has been no parallel movement supporting men in redefining masculinity in a healthy, modern context.

A meta-analysis by Wong et al. (2017), reviewing 78 studies, found that rigid adherence to traditional masculine norms is associated with poorer mental health. However, when certain masculine traits like leadership, strength, and responsibility are embraced with flexibility and intention, they can enhance psychological well-being. Masculinity itself is not harmful; rather, it is the unexamined extremes and rigidity that become damaging.

It is worth noting that some therapeutic approaches, particularly feminist viewpoints, might emphasise different aspects of this dynamic, focusing more on dismantling patriarchal structures rather than reclaiming positive masculinity. Both perspectives offer valuable insights, though my clinical experience suggests that approaches affirming healthy masculine traits alongside help-seeking and emotional expression tend to be more effective with male clients.

Beyond Stoicism: The Double Bind of Modern Masculinity

This is supported by studies that show traditional gender roles for men, such as being providers and protectors themselves, are not harmful, and can offer purpose and identity when fulfilled responsibly and ethically. However, when enforced rigidly, they may discourage emotional expression and help-seeking in men. Chan and Hayashi (2010) found that cultural expectations of stoicism can harm men's mental health.

This demonstrates why we need a more flexible understanding of masculinity. The issue is not with traditional roles themselves, but rather with the rigid belief that emotional expression signifies weakness or failure. To avoid being perceived this way, many men remain silent and suppress their feelings, leading to isolated suffering and deteriorating mental health.

However, there is a concerning trend emerging on the opposite end of the spectrum, insisting men must openly express emotions or risk being labelled as "emotionally unavailable" or "emotionally immature." Men should not be forced into a new form of emotional rigidity (i.e., *having* to express all emotions publicly) but should have safe spaces to explore and share them authentically.

Recommendations for Healthy Masculinity Development

1. **Create safe spaces** for boys and men to explore and define masculinity without shame or rigid expectations.
2. **Educate** on terms like 'toxic masculinity' and 'narcissism' to prevent misuse, mislabelling, and stigma.
3. **Affirm healthy traits** such as leadership, responsibility, and emotional resilience across homes, schools, and workplaces.
4. **Reframe traditional roles** like providing and protecting by also valuing emotional connection, care, and promoting role models who embody both strength and vulnerability.

3. Redefining Success: Character Beyond Currency

Society measures success like a balance sheet, reducing worth to money, status, and appearance. But men say their fathers - present in body but absent in heart - taught them the opposite lesson.

Degrees and achievements can open doors, but they cannot sustain meaningful relationships or lifelong fulfilment. Whilst success is often measured by salary, strength, or accolades, true legacy lies in character, in how a man shows up, stays present, and leads with integrity. Despite this, many men carry a silent fear of judgment and failure, one that pushes them to constantly prove their worth through external measures. A man's sense of worth is healthier when it is rooted internally, shaped by identity, purpose, and values, not by validation from status or performance.

The Pressure of Performance

Men today are bombarded with narrow definitions of success: physical strength, status, and wealth. Society tells them that value is earned through accumulation and appearance. Many of my clients express the relentless pressure to achieve, often chasing ideals they never chose. But when they reflect on their fathers, men who "had it all" but remained emotionally distant, a deeper wisdom emerges; real success is about emotional presence and integrity, not just material gain.

Despite this, peer pressure and social media often reinforce a harmful message that happiness and success are defined by income and popularity. These influences are strong but misaligned with what truly matters, a truth many men come to understand through therapy. While psychological frameworks highlight the benefits of achievement and goal-setting, relying solely on external success as the basis for identity and self-worth can ultimately harm mental and emotional well-being.

What Men Value in Their Fathers

I meet men who deeply appreciate their fathers' hard work, yet carry emotional wounds from absence, inconsistency, or lack of vulnerability. Their reflections speak volumes:

> *"I appreciated my father's hard work, but I just wanted him to spend more time with me."*
> *"I would have respected him more if he treated my mother with kindness."*
> *"I didn't need my dad to be rich, I needed him to be reliable and ask me how I was feeling."*

> "*My father cared more about his new girlfriend/wife than he cared about me.*"
> "*My father never talked about his feelings.*" and
> "*I hardly saw my dad; he was always at work.*"

These statements reveal a truth: children, especially sons, remember not what their fathers earned, but how they showed up. This clinical insight aligns with Seligman's (2011) research on authentic happiness, which shows that a sense of purpose and meaningful relationships are stronger predictors of life satisfaction than financial success.

Men often reflect on the kind of man they wish their father had been, or the kind they hope to become. Time and again, the same qualities surface:

- *Honesty and Integrity* – Living in alignment with one's values. Many men describe the peace that comes from letting go of external validation and showing up as their authentic selves.
- *Reliability and Consistency* – Whether it's picking up children on time or supporting a friend through a crisis, reliability builds trust.
- *Emotional Strength* – Not stoicism, but the courage to be present, stay calm in conflict, and engage with vulnerability.
- *Protectiveness* – Creating emotionally, mentally, and physically safe spaces at home, at work, and in relationships.
- *Provision* – Beyond financial support, provision includes emotional presence, practical care, and dependability.
- *Supportiveness* – Being available to offer help, emotional or practical. These small acts create a foundation of connection and security.

Redefining Success: Where True Wealth Lives

Messages about self-worth begin early. A father who only acknowledges accomplishments, a mother who constantly compares, or a teacher who shames instead of supports can plant deep beliefs:

> *"I'm only worthy if I achieve."*
> *"I must be perfect to be loved."* or
> *"If I fail, I'm worthless."*

These narratives often follow men for decades. When I ask male clients what success means to them, the initial answers are predictable: "a good job" and "a good income". But as we explore deeper, it becomes clear these were never truly their definitions. They were inherited, absorbed from culture, family, or peers, rarely questioned, but deeply internalised. For many men, especially those reflecting on fatherhood or healing from strained paternal bonds, what matters most is not status or wealth, but sincerity, emotional availability, and genuine presence. Emotional connection leaves a far richer mark than material success.

Redefining success means shifting the focus from what a man earns to how he lives, how he loves, and how he shows up for others and himself. Beyond that, no matter what success looks like, men need to feel safe to speak about their struggles of trying to achieve and succeed without shame or judgment. From a young age, showing emotion and asking for help must be seen as signs of courage, not weakness. This vulnerability creates space for authenticity, connection, and growth throughout their lives.

Today's men have the opportunity to model a fuller definition of success, one that values character alongside currency. While achievement and financial success have their place, leading with presence, honesty, and emotional courage allows us to break harmful generational patterns and offer the next generation something far more lasting than wealth: a grounded sense of what it truly means to be a man, in fact, to be human.

Recommendations for Character-Based Success

1. **Promote core traits**: honesty, emotional strength, reliability, protectiveness, supportiveness, and care.
2. **Reimagine education**: include life skills, emotional literacy, practical intelligence, and real-world problem-solving.
3. **Mentorship**: connect boys with male mentors who show character, and purpose-driven leadership in school, work, and life.
4. **Support self-reflection**: help boys and men challenge old ideas of success and set authentic, value-driven goals.

Conclusion: Breaking the Code

This chapter explores the idea of breaking the code, challenging false beliefs, and unlearning harmful ideas about self-worth, masculinity, and success that pressure men to conform and suffer in silence.

Understanding men's mental health requires examining early experiences and the social messages that shape boys as they grow into men. From a young age, many boys are judged by narrow external standards while their emotional needs are overlooked. Consequently, they learn to suppress vulnerability, internalising the message that showing emotion is a sign of weakness. This often leads to low self-esteem, increased anxiety and depression, emotional isolation, and difficulties in relationships.

Healthy self-esteem begins with consistent emotional nurturing. Boys need encouragement to work hard and aim high, but they must also know that their worth is not defined by grades, trophies, or outcomes. Parents, teachers, and other adults play a vital role in delivering this message. Without it, boys may begin to seek validation through constant performance and perfection, chasing ideals that are often unrealistic and unsustainable.

Masculinity needs to be redefined, not rejected. Men deserve the freedom and safety to shape their own understanding of what it means to be a man, just as women have increasingly been able to shape their own roles. The traditional demand for silence and stoicism is harmful. Boys should be encouraged to speak openly, show emotion, and ask for help without fear of judgment. Whether they are preparing for exams, playing sport, facing challenges in relationships, or dealing with pressure at work, seeking support must be seen as strength, not weakness.

When the fear of judgement and failure learned in childhood follows boys into adulthood, it often silences them at the very moments they most need help. In careers, in relationships, and in fatherhood, this silence can be damaging. Yet research shows that resilience is not built by avoiding failure, but by facing it, learning from it, and adapting.

To truly support men, we must challenge narrow definitions of success and create environments where they are encouraged to strive, but also to be emotionally seen and heard. This involves teaching that self-worth is grounded in values, not performance. It means showing that masculinity can include vulnerability, openness, and compassion. It means redefining success not in terms of money, status, or appearance, but through character, connection, and authenticity.

Breaking the code does not mean rejecting achievement, whether in academics, sports, music, or work. Nor does it mean dismissing traditional or modern forms of masculinity. Rather, it's about redefining all of these through courage, compassion, and emotional honesty. Whether it's a boy navigating exam pressure or a man balancing life's demands, we must empower them to know: expressing emotions, asking for help, and showing vulnerability are not just acceptable—they are acts of true courage.

Dedication: Celebrating The Heart of Men

I have experienced genuine love and beauty in men. The ones who leave the deepest mark are those with the kindest hearts, who stay when times are hardest, who say *"sorry"* and *"thank you"* with true humility, and who love beyond the bounds of romance.

These men remind me of the true grace and power of masculinity:

The father who didn't raise you like a *princess*, but like an *empress*, worthy of honor. The brother who carries all the weight without ever complaining. The son who reads your face and asks how you are, and often. The client who expresses, without hesitation, words of utmost respect and appreciation. And above all, the beloved friend whose unconditional love and silent presence nourished your soul, and whose memory still does. *(This chapter was written in honor of just such a friend.)*

In my experience, what women remember most about men is not their achievements or status, but how they made us feel safe, seen, and appreciated. That is a true legacy, one that remains long after they are gone.

So, to the men out there, we value your intrinsic worth, and the world needs you now, more than ever!

Final Reflection: What Being a Therapist Taught Me

People often ask me, "*Doesn't it affect you, listening to people's problems all the time?*" The answer is, of course, it does—this is how it has affected me, and these are the truths I hope my own sons come to know.

After bearing witness to thousands upon thousands of stories of suffering, trauma, healing, and the unrelenting human search for meaning, I have come to understand a few insights that cut across every walk of life, gender, race, and status.

True success is not measured by the wealth in our bank accounts, but by the compassion in our hearts and our steady commitment to justice.

Money and status may draw attention for a moment, but they cannot define our essence. When the spotlight fades and fortunes slip away, we discover what remains: how we made others feel. In the end, and in silence, we are all faced with the same questions: *Did we lift others up, or did we push them down? Did we stand for what was right when it mattered most? And did we leave the people around us better than we found them?*

Ultimately, our identity isn't defined by what we own, but who we choose to be when there is no audience, how we carry ourselves when power is in our hands, and how we treat those who have nothing to offer us in return; that's our character. A life built on integrity, kindness, and honesty will outlast any monument. It leaves behind something more enduring: a quiet, profound respect that echoes through generations. Kingdoms crumble and fortunes scatter like dust in the wind, but a soul that cares deeply and gives freely lives on in ways that no amount of material wealth ever could.*

---

* **Bibliography**

Carlson, R. W., & Fishbach, A. (2024). Learning from failure: The roles of self-focused feedback, task expectations, and subsequent instruction. *Journal of Experimental Psychology: General*, 153(5), 1025–1045. https://doi.org/10.1037/xge0001078

Chan, R. K. H., & Hayashi, K. (2010). *Gender roles and help-seeking behaviour: Promoting professional help among Japanese men*. Journal of Social Work, 10(3), 243–262.

Dweck, C. S. (2006). *Mindset: The new psychology of success*. Random House.

Gerdes, Z. T., Levant, R. F., & Jadaszewski, S. (2021). A systematic review of the relationship between conformity to masculine norms and mental health among men. *Psychology of Men & Masculinities*, 22(1), 76-90.

Kiselica, M. S., & Englar-Carlson, M. (2010). Identifying, affirming, and building upon male strengths: The positive psychology/positive masculinity model of psychotherapy with boys and men. *Psychotherapy: Theory, Research, Practice, Training*, 47(3), 276-287.

Levant, R. F., & Richmond, K. (2016). The gender role strain paradigm and masculinity ideologies. In Y. J. Wong & S. R. Wester (Eds.), *APA handbook of men and masculinities* (pp. 23-49). American Psychological Association.

Seligman, M. E. P. (2011). *Flourish: A visionary new understanding of happiness and well-being*. Free Press.

Wong, Y. J., Ho, M. H. R., Wang, S. Y., & Miller, I. S. K. (2017). Meta-analyses of the relationship between conformity to masculine norms and mental health-related outcomes. *Journal of Counseling Psychology*, 64(1), 80-93.

ABOUT the AUTHOR

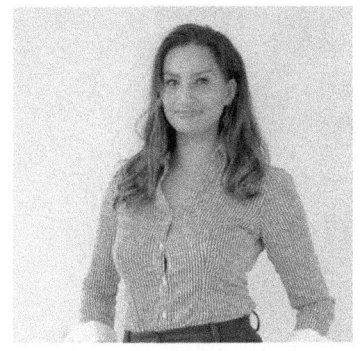

Roje Khalique is a clinical consultant and founder of rkTherapy, a London-based psychology service delivering culturally intelligent therapy for high-achieving professionals. With 20 years in mental health, she specialises in supporting both men and women with depression and a wide range of anxiety disorders.

Roje offers bespoke one-to-one therapy and online group psycho-coaching, including London in-person intensives. She works with clients in the U.K., U.S., the Middle East, and Asia. Roje created *Anxiet-Ease: Therapy In Your Hands®*, a digital Cognitive Behavioural Therapy (CBT) guided self-help training.

Social Link:
linktr.ee/rkhalique

Chapter 10

A Paradigm Shift in Men's Mental Health

Dr. Stacey Kevin Frick

"Most men lead lives of quiet desperation."

— Henry David Thoreau

I can't remember what he said to insult me, but I do remember the adrenaline coursing through my veins as I walked towards him.

No one was going to talk to me like that. I had spent my childhood being terrorized by a father who believed that the more shit I could take, mentally and physically, the manlier I'd become, and that twisted belief planted a deep root in my psyche.

"Get out of the car," I said.

Then he reached under the seat for a gun.

Everything stopped.

The noise in my head. The fury in my body. The illusion of control.

In that instant, I realized I wasn't just walking toward a fight. I could be walking toward my death. And for what? Ego? Pride? A false sense of power? That moment didn't just break me open; it exposed the lie I had been living. My entire definition of what it meant to be a man was warped. And it almost got me killed.

That was the beginning of a shift that would take years to unfold.

You see, we've been lied to. We've been told that real men don't back down, don't feel pain, don't talk about their emotions. We've been handed a blueprint built on silence and suppression, and then punished when that silence explodes.

But it doesn't have to be this way.

For centuries, the idea of masculinity has been built on an unwavering image of strength, resilience, dominance, and silent suffering. Men have been conditioned to be the protectors, the providers, the ones who "tough it out" through every challenge life throws at them. This conditioning has created a systemic stigma, bias, and limiting belief system, culturally placed, that opposes men's mental health. In this relentless pursuit of societal expectations, something has been lost: the acknowledgment that men, too, are emotional beings with an inherent need for mental well-being.

The truth is that mental health is not a sign of weakness. It is an indication of strength. When men allow themselves to embrace emotional awareness and self-reflection, they unlock a power far greater than physical strength or external achievements. They gain the ability to lead more fulfilling lives, build healthier relationships, and cultivate a sense of self that is not bound by outdated stereotypes.

From an early age, boys are taught that expressing vulnerability is a sign of weakness and failure. We are told to *man up*, that *boys don't cry, don't be so sensitive*, and to *walk it off*. Social expectations condemn emotions that don't fit into the narrow definitions of masculinity. Strength is equated with aggression, power, and virility. Emotional repression becomes a rite of passage. Over time, these rigid constructs create an internal battle—one that many men fight in silence.

Society has long romanticized the image of the tortured, burdened man. Struggle and pain are normalized and worn proudly as a badge of courage and evidence of resilience. We tell men that they must push through hardships alone, that seeking help is a betrayal of their masculinity. The focus is on the wounds they carry and on them being damaged, rather than seeing opportunities for growth and expansion.

I remember when I was 31 years old, applying for a medical insurance policy. I am a non-smoker, non-drinker, and avid gym rat. I did not qualify for the top-tier coverage. *REALLY?!?!* I was so confused as to why, so I started looking into it. My application stated "mental nervousness" as the reason. I did some digging and found out that the insurance company had taken the information that I had worked with a mental health professional, and, without ever having a diagnosis of "mental nervousness" in my record, they used this as a weakness against me. I was unceremoniously victimized for prioritizing my mental health.

This is just one example of how systematically we are told that mental health care is bad. I thought about this more and applied it to other areas of my life. I didn't see anywhere on my application where, because I worked with a personal trainer, they labeled me "out of shape," nor did I see anyone labeling me at a bank as "not good with money" because I use a financial advisor. Nobody is eager to single me out as a "sinner" if I go to a house of worship. Why do we stigmatize mental health in this way and not any other form of health, be it financial, physical, or spiritual? The American Psychological Association (APA) has identified traditional masculine norms as: risk-taking, dominance, emotional control, and the primacy of work over personal well-being. While these traits can sometimes serve a purpose, they often lead to severe consequences: depression, stress, body image issues, substance abuse, and difficulty forming healthy relationships. The expectation to constantly perform, provide, and protect leaves little room for self-care or emotional expression.

This unrelenting pressure leads to increased stress, mental health challenges, and an aversion to seeking help. Studies show that men are far less likely than women to reach out for professional support, leading to unhealthy coping mechanisms such as substance abuse, isolation, or destructive behaviors.

However, the good news is that this cycle is not inevitable. (Thankfully!) It is a choice. A choice to redefine masculinity, to embrace mental health as a strength, and to recognize that true power comes not from suppression, but from expansion.

Mental health is not just about healing wounds—it is about growing, expanding, and improving. Just as a well-equipped toolbox allows a craftsman to build and repair with precision, prioritizing mental health provides men with the tools to navigate life's challenges more effectively.

For too long, the traits associated with traditional masculinity—physical toughness, aggression, independence, and emotional restraint—have been seen as the only tools available. These traits are not inherently negative; they serve a purpose and can be extremely powerful. But they are not the only tools men have available. Growth means adding to the toolbox, not discarding what already exists.

Mental health is a tool that collects other tools. Imagine mental health as a tool belt. My father was a carpenter, among other things, and I remember vividly how his tool belt held his tools so perfectly. With mental health as your tool belt, you can now add many other tools to use in life. The beauty of this tool belt is that it is never full. You never lose any of the tools that you have gathered previously. You only add new tools.

Imagine a man who has spent his entire life relying on brute strength to solve problems. What happens when he encounters a challenge that requires patience, emotional intelligence, or self-compassion? Without these additional tools, he is left struggling. But when he allows himself to develop these skills, he not only still has all of the strength he had before, but he also becomes adaptable, resilient, and better equipped to handle any situation life throws his way.

Men are far more than the rigid stereotypes imposed upon them. We are dynamic, multifaceted beings capable of incredible growth, kindness, and wisdom.

Consider the scholar-athlete: a man who excels both intellectually and physically, embodying a balance of strength and knowledge. Or the benevolent leader, whose power is rooted in wisdom and compassion rather than dominance and control. These examples illustrate that masculinity is not a one-size-fits-all concept—it is a spectrum of experiences, strengths, and attributes that evolve over time.

I did not always prioritize my mental health, and it shows in the story of my life. The tools that I had were simple and primitive, and I used them to the best of my abilities. However, when I began taking care of my mental health, I saw incredible changes. In every aspect of my life as a doctor, a CEO leading a company, a romantic partner, and a friend, the tools I was able to add and use made me a better man. They made me a better person.

In fact, leaning into my own mental well-being saved me from living a life that was in no way aligned with my true nature. You see, I was a veterinarian by trade and went on to build and become the CEO of a multi-hospital system. I had way more money than I needed, the hot cars, multiple homes, the jet-set life. On paper, I was a huge success story and had achieved goals most people put on their vision boards. It doesn't get much more manly than that!

And I was miserable.

I realized that the clock was ticking and that none of the material things were resulting in any kind of happiness. So, I did something that made most of the people in my life question my sanity. I sold everything. I quit running the hospitals and started my company, The Empowerment Revolution. My mission was to help as many people as possible rewrite the inner codes that were programmed in their childhood and throughout their history, and were now making them miserable as adults.

We all have running codes that inform our choices and our results. The problem is that most of those codes were installed years ago. Some codes we installed after listening to people who might have meant well, but we installed programs that made *them* comfortable. We learned about love, masculinity, pride, and success from people we trusted, and now it's time to question if the programs we installed match the life we actually want to live.

Men's mental health is not about conforming to a specific or outdated mold but rather embracing our unique identity and recognizing that our emotional well-being is just as important as any other aspect of our lives. It's about empowering men to walk their own path and to embrace their empathy and their emotions, not as a bridge to being soft, but as a bridge to being real. To being human. To being the kind of person others feel safe with.

The journey toward redefining masculinity and mental health is not about discarding the past but about evolving beyond its limitations. We don't lose who we are when we prioritize mental health; we gain a greater understanding of ourselves. We find more confidence in our journey and less influence from societal idols. The money, fame, power, and pleasure that we are told are motivations and goals become consequences of our service and impact. Real strength is having the ability to rule your kingdom with fear, violence, anger, and dominance, then choosing not to. When you have the tools that mental health provides, you can choose the ones that will display emotional maturity and result in respect, sustainability, and trust.

We must frame mental health as a tool for self-improvement rather than as a sign of deficiency. Just as physical fitness is celebrated as a means of strength, mental well-being should be viewed in the same light. There is no shame in seeking help, in developing emotional intelligence, or in practicing self-care. These actions do not diminish a man's strength—they enhance it.

If we are to truly create change, we must normalize and celebrate men who prioritize their mental health. We must dismantle the outdated beliefs that perpetuate stigma and replace them with a culture of compassion and understanding.

This starts with each of us. We must challenge our own biases, offer grace to ourselves and others, and create spaces where men feel safe to express themselves without fear of judgment. When we support men in their mental health journey, we empower them to live fully, freely, and authentically.

I remember when the only tools in life that I had were anger, physical strength, and a state of lack. I believed that if I could hold the hot coal the longest, I would be able to achieve my goals. When I gave my mental health precedence, I found that not only did I have all the tools at my disposal that worked before, but I also gathered new tools that made my challenges different. They became less difficult. My goals changed. I started cooperating with life instead of fighting it. When I put energy into my mental health, I didn't become *less* in any area. I did not become physically weaker, less respected, less effective, or less of a man. Just the opposite. I became physically stronger and arguably "tougher", but I never got into physical altercations anymore. I became more respected for having a level head and being easier to communicate with. I became more effective in so many areas of my life. I was able to embrace my life in new, amazing ways, and in doing so, allowed a reality that is more beautiful than I ever could have imagined.

When mental health is cared for, all the tools in the tool belt are implemented in a way that creates our highest greatness. We empower ourselves and those that we encounter. We stand confident in our choices and courageous in the face of our vulnerability.

It is time to move beyond the quiet desperation that Thoreau spoke of and into a new era—one where mental health is recognized not as a weakness, but as the ultimate strength.

To learn more www.drstaceykevinfrick.com

ABOUT the AUTHOR

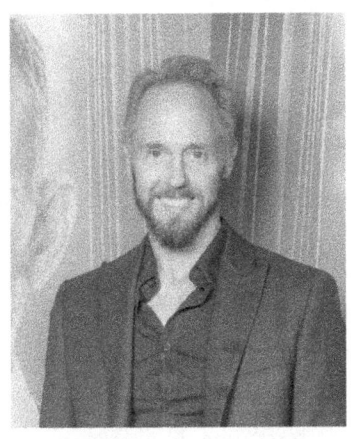

Dr. Stacey Kevin Frick is a seasoned leader and visionary dedicated to fostering health, well-being, and financial empowerment. After practicing medicine for over 20 years and serving as CEO of multiple successful businesses, Dr. Frick now dedicates his life to empowering others to lead a life of fulfillment and impact. His mission is to guide individuals toward lives and businesses to create joy, abundance, and purpose, grounded in authenticity and personal empowerment.

As a best-selling author, speaker, and founder of The Empowerment Revolution, Dr. Frick merges his extensive leadership expertise and business acumen with holistic well-being practices to create transformative pathways for success. A highly sought-after keynote speaker, author, and entrepreneur, he specializes in boosting self-confidence, enhancing emotional intelligence, and fostering personal growth. His passion for helping individuals overcome personal and professional barriers defines his career and legacy.

Dr. Frick's journey reflects a multifaceted soul with a deep commitment to knowledge, leadership, and innovation. Beyond his professional accomplishments, he finds inspiration in literature, the arts, and fitness, continually enriching his understanding of the world. His dedication to mental health, holistic healing, alternative medicine, and nutrition demonstrates his unwavering belief in the power of a balanced and health-focused lifestyle.

Through his work, Dr. Frick provides a beacon of inspiration and guidance for those seeking financial abundance, holistic well-being, and a deeper connection to their authentic selves. His leadership exemplifies the transformative power of service, offering tools and motivation to those ready to embark on a journey of growth and self-discovery.

Whether you aspire to professional success, improved health, or a more meaningful life, Dr. Stacey Kevin Frick stands as a trusted guide and mentor. His life's mission is to inspire and transform others, helping them unlock their full potential and embrace a future filled with purpose and fulfillment.

Social Links

www.linkedin.com/in/dr-stacey-kevin-frick-8b13614/
www.instagram.com/staceykevinfrick/
www.facebook.com/stacey.k.frick
amazon.com/author/drstaceykevinfrick

Chapter 11

Such a Heavy Load

Steven A. Schechter

Every time I see my first-grade picture, the time travel is instantaneous. I remember sitting on the front porch one day, holding my knees tightly to my chest. I was wearing my blue suit for first-grade picture day. It was Friday, February 8, 1974, and my parents' divorce was finally official. The court awarded my mother full custody, but my father could still see us. He had to come to pick us up every other Saturday morning and bring us home the following Sunday night in time for dinner.

Back at my mother's, I'd put the groceries away, but never in the right place. Or I'd fold the clothes, but they wouldn't fit in the drawers right...she always doled out the chastisement, full of condescension. I was six years old, wondering why my mother didn't love me anymore. She couldn't forgive my grandfather, she couldn't forgive my father, and now she couldn't forgive me for reminding her of them.

Since my dad was gone, my mother didn't have anywhere else to direct her anger toward my grandfather, so I got it. No matter what I did, she was never happy with what I did...I could never be good enough. Procrastination and perfectionism set in, and I became a people pleaser. The narcissist had complete control, and I felt crushed and unloved.

My mother struggled with her weight her entire life. After my younger brother was born, the baby weight didn't come off. My father was genuinely concerned about her health because the following three years resulted in a weight gain of 120 pounds for her.

"Candy, don't you think 40 pounds a year is a problem? Shouldn't we seek help?" he asked.

She heard what she had been hearing throughout her entire life: "You're fat."

"Ian, I want a divorce," she replied.

After the divorce, my mom lost all the weight. At one point, her 5'2" frame weighed 110 pounds. Cigarettes didn't do enough to curb her appetite, so bulimia took over. She started smoking pot with her boyfriend, using a bong she disguised as a flower vase. They had a fight, and she couldn't forgive him. She stopped sticking her finger down her throat, and things started getting worse.

Seven years later, 110 pounds had become three hundred. At this point, my grandmother started making all her clothes. I'm 13 years of age at this point and have the same worries my dad did about my mom. I gathered up my courage and asked my mom what I could do to help. Well, I did the wrong thing again.

"If I have to talk to one more person about my weight one more time, I'm going to kill myself!" This time, she didn't pick me apart, criticize me, or minimize me; she psychologically manipulated me. I was devastated, terrified, and became the six-year-old boy again, sitting on the porch in my blue suit, clutching my knees to my chest, and wondering why my mother didn't love me anymore. The crime I committed was caring for my mom. I needed someone to talk to, but had no one. Yeah, I got to see my dad every two weeks, but I couldn't talk to him because our visits were too fun and too short. The same went for seeing my grandparents, Bam and Papa, on Friday nights. My reward was isolation and loneliness. The weight was too much to bear.

To understand a narcissist, imagine someone who is like a black hole of self-importance. This person sucks all the air out of the room, making everything about him or herself. This person is a master of manipulation who uses charm and guilt to get what he or she wants and never apologizes because this person is always right. Dealing with a narcissist is like fighting a shadow. You can't win because the narcissist twists everything around to make you the villain. So, self-defense is the key. We'll talk more about that later.

Two years later, I was sitting in ninth-grade Spanish. I badly wanted recognition for an accomplishment or to be offered an opportunity. I was daydreaming about going to the principal's office for recognition when something brought me back to reality.

Knock, knock, knock.

"Steve," my teacher said. "The principal wants you in his office."

When I turned the corner and stepped into the main corridor to the front of the school, there was my mom. My heart dropped; I just knew…my dad was dead.

My brother and I hadn't seen him in a month because he had to cancel our visit two weeks ago to cover a shift for a stupid no-show at work. Seven days later was his funeral, March 19, 1982. Soon after, I remember curling up on the couch with his bowling ball, crying next to my mom. She offered no comfort. Now I felt underwater, and the bowling ball had become an anchor.

When I went to college, it was incredible to be free and dream about becoming an electrical engineer. Driving away lifted a great deal of weight off my shoulders even as my mother stood on the steps by herself, crying. I made new friends and took interesting classes. Then the results of my first semester arrived. Learning that I wasn't near the top of my class anymore stunned me. In fact, I was average. This left me deflated again. I struggled to climb out of that hole.

Just when I felt like I had traction, my mom got t-boned in an intersection on her way to work, a mile from our house. She walked away from that with a broken ankle, a total loss on her Oldsmobile Regency, a medical disability, and retirement. Helping her deal with that took enough effort that I missed half of a semester; a four-year engineering degree became six.

On top of that, the job market sucked. No one was having luck landing a job interview, let alone a job. I was at my wits' end, so I had one choice remaining – the Army Corps of Engineers. It was two weeks before graduation, and despite setbacks in the application process, I was the first student in my class to land a job in research and development (R&D).

One Monday morning that same year, Vicki, an R&D assistant, walks over and asks, "Steve, are you single?" I had just broken up with my girlfriend on Friday, so "Yes, I am."

The next day, Vicki bops down the aisle with a friend. "Hi Steve. This is Laura. Laura's single. Laura, this is Steve. Steve's single." I watched the embarrassment climb up Laura's neck and into her face like a thermometer. They scurried away and giggled like schoolgirls.

The next day, Vicki swung by my cubicle again. "So, Steve, what do you think? Did you like Laura?" she asked.

"Yeah, she seemed nice," I said.

"Would you ask her out on a date?" she asked. "Sure, I'd ask her out."

Vicki pressed on, "How's Thursday at Cactus Grille around noon sound?

"Um, OK, I guess." It only took one date, and I was floating.

My family was small while Laura's was huge. The best wedding advice we received was from my grandmother, Bam. *Never go to bed mad.* It's been 32 years, and we still heed her advice. After growing up with a narcissist, Bam's wedding advice was the first mention I'd heard of forgiveness.

The first couple of years were great as long as we didn't have a disagreement. When we did have one, it was startling. In my house, raising your voice was a sin. In Laura's, the only way someone heard you above the din was to raise your voice. I was quiet while she slammed doors.

"What did I get myself into?" I wondered. We decided we needed to learn how to fight fairly. The tool we learned in marriage counseling was to never have anything between us when we worked through a problem. This meant no furniture, no sitting across the room from each other, no pillows, nothing. We had to sit directly across from each other, hold hands, and touch knees. Knowing we were each just as vulnerable as the other was a complete game-changer. This was my second lesson about forgiveness.

Fifteen years later, on my commute from Jamestown, a car passed me at a narrow point in the road right before a curve and knocked me off the road. Flight for Life flew me to Denver with two cracks in my skull, two cracked ribs, and a broken left collarbone. The first thing I remember was six days later. G-d** had many angels watching over me that day. If some of G-d's greatest gifts are unanswered prayers, why did He answer this one?

During one of my physical therapy sessions, my therapist became uncharacteristically quiet. "What's wrong?" I asked.

"You don't know how lucky you are, sweetie," she replied.

"Oh, but I do; an EMT found me, a second rider brought back an ambulance, Flight for Life, and five broken bones."

"No, honey. You don't understand," she said. "Let me explain what is going on with your left shoulder. Do you feel here, where I'm working on the place where your neck meets your left shoulder?" she asked. I nodded my head.

"This is where the blood pooled from your head injury. In my 20 years of working with TBI (traumatic brain injury) patients, you are the only one who isn't a quadriplegic."

Now I'm the quiet one. And ashen. Things are suddenly a little out of focus. I had just learned to be careful what I ask for; G-d just might answer my prayers.

Forty percent of couples' marriages do not survive a traumatic brain injury. Now you understand why we made it. Laura knew before I did about my crash. In fact, when it happened, she was there spiritually. I lay there close to death, and she talked me down off the ledge. I didn't realize how close we truly were. At that moment, Laura was the best thing that ever happened to me. Again. I grew up in a broken

---

* In Judaism, all books with G-d's name are holy. These books cannot be burned or thrown away if they become damaged. Instead, they must be buried in a special ceremony. All Jewish cemeteries have an area where they bury these damaged books, usually once a year. Spelling G-d's name in this way keeps the book from becoming holy; if it is ruined then there is no disrespect to Him resulting from that ruinous act.

house without religion, had no faith, and hadn't attended a service in 41 years. Suddenly, it was time to go to church with Laura and the kids.

I started attending Catholic Mass with my family in 2009. I learned the songs and the prayers said during mass, put G-d in place of Jesus, and I started talking to G-d again. Our kids were no longer going to Catholic school because my son's third-grade teacher bullied him, so we put them in religious education (RE) at our new church. We made great friends there. It was exciting to have others want my Jewish perspective. We had fun with everyone learning that we called our kids *cashews* (Catholic Jews).

While I was loving my spiritual awakening, work was another issue. It took us two years to qualify for a mortgage while we lived with Laura's parents. Between that, the business we lost, and the other jobs I had, key people I worked with were so selfish and egotistical.

I had this nagging question in my mind: *How do you seek help when the one person you were supposed to have trusted the most in your youth made you carry their burden?* It was a question I'd been unable to answer for over 50 years. A new therapist helped me see that my mom was the first narcissist in my life. Every job and business venture I had after getting my MBA had brought me face to face with the same person: her. I realized that the key people in my business life had been narcissists as well.

We are all here to learn what G-d wants to teach us. If we don't pass the test, the next lesson will be harder. For me, that lesson was dealing with gaslighting. Gaslighting is a form of psychological manipulation where someone makes another person question their own sanity, memories, or perceptions of reality. It's a type of emotional abuse that can lead to confusion, anxiety, and even mental health issues like anxiety, depression, and post-traumatic stress disorder (PTSD).

The most recent narcissist, Will, wielded this kind of abuse for two years before I realized what occurred. He modified my work to make others believe that I was unable to do decent work. He would say things only to me while telling a different story to everyone else. By the time he finished with me, the only person at that job who mattered to me believed that I made no contributions and that Will had done it all. I gave everything to this company and received "firing without cause" as a reward.

After that, I didn't work for a long time. Instead, all I did was argue with Will in my head about my worth, and I never won. I concluded that I had no value, couldn't get any job because he had gaslit me for so long that the only thing I thought I could be was the lonely six-year-old on the front porch again. Will was living in my head rent-free, and I felt hopeless. No matter what I did, he and the other narcissists were always there. I felt doomed to hopelessly live in this never-ending cycle of rumination.

Thankfully, Laura was still by my side. She learned about eye movement desensitization and reprocessing (EMDR) and convinced me that it was time to go back to therapy. The therapist used EMDR therapy to throw me a proverbial flotation device. I was bobbing and sinking, so I grabbed onto it with all that I had. EMDR is a form of psychotherapy designed to treat post-traumatic stress disorder (PTSD). EMDR aims to reduce subjective distress and strengthen adaptive beliefs related to traumatic events. It develops new neural pathways in the brain to create new habits to replace conclusions from traumatic events with new frames of reference with which to develop healthier conclusions. That EMDR therapist gave me my life back.

My biggest takeaway from therapy was how to defend myself against a narcissist. While it is still challenging for me, I've learned that with the right strategies, I can protect my mental and emotional well-being. Here is a set of effective self-defense techniques I learned and offer up for you to consider:

1. Set clear boundaries. Define your limits and stick to your guns.
2. Don't take it personally. It's not about you; it's about them.
3. Limit emotional engagement. Avoid their drama by using indifferent responses that reduce their power over you.

4. Practice assertive communication. Use "I" statements to express your feelings and needs without blaming them. For example, say, "I feel uncomfortable when..." instead of, "You always..."
5. Be direct and concise. A narcissist can twist or manipulate lengthy explanations.
6. Understand narcissism. Better recognize manipulation tactics and strengthen your appropriate responses.
7. Surround yourself with supportive people.
8. Consider professional help. Prioritize your well-being.
9. Practice mindfulness: deep breathing and meditation reduce stress and keep you grounded.
10. Know when to walk away.

Since I couldn't depend on my mother, I spent my entire life doing everything for myself. Everything was about me. I attached my identity to what I did, not who I was. With that came pride in accomplishments that I thought were my own making. A life full of pride led me to pray to the wrong god. I had put myself ahead of G-d. I never thanked Him for the good things in life, but was good at yelling, "Alright already!" to Him when things didn't go the way I wanted. An old piece of Yiddish advice asks, *Do you want to make G-d laugh? Tell Him your plans.* Boy, does He laugh at me.

My therapist helped me understand that I had transferred my feelings about my mom onto God, which kept me from counting on Him. I was never good enough for my mother, so I was never good enough for Him either. I had to perform to earn love and approval from everyone in my life, the curse of a people pleaser. I got to the point where I felt I deserved nothing, and I could not open my heart to G-d. This left me not understanding G-d's unconditional love. I went through life unable to lean into that love of His and trust Him. I learned to seek validation from everyone and everything *but* G-d by attaching my identity to what I did instead of who I was. It doesn't matter how many antidepressants and anxiety medications you take because there aren't enough in the world to make narcissism, procrastination, perfectionism, and depression go away.

When my daughter was 16, she told us how she had been bullied in elementary Catholic school because I was Jewish. I was angry, lost, and sad because, of all places, this should not occur in a Catholic school. Since this was a behavior her classmates learned from their parents, I lost the tether anchoring me to the church, and so did she. Since Bam had passed away years ago, I became weighed down with having no roots in my Jewish faith. I felt that I had no one to talk to again.

The loss of my Jewish roots left me floating until I found a new *shul*. After I attended my first service, I felt better. A month later, I crossed paths with my rabbi at the store and went back for my second service. Six weeks after that, while struggling with Will having just fired me, I received a text from Rabbi unexpectedly. It couldn't have come at a better time. I was sinking and couldn't get back up, so I went to *shul* that Saturday and felt as if I had finally come home. Others introduced themselves to me, and whichever direction I turned, I fit in. I finally had an answer to the deeper question that had plagued me during my entire, narcissistic-filled life: "Do I really matter?"

"Yes!" G-d replied.

I've been to *shul* every Saturday and every holiday since. A wonderful book, *On Purpose*, by Mendel Kalmenson, helped me finally understand why I am here. I've learned that every action I take, no matter how small, holds enormous potential. Since I matter, everything I do matters. Every encounter that I have may be the most important opportunity in my life. Hence, every time I help someone else, it is the most important thing that I will ever do. That interaction may be the exact reason G-d put me here. Once I finish, it may be my last effort here on Earth.

Today, my relationship with G-d is what defines me. Instead of being angry with someone because they don't do what I think they should do, now I understand that it's all about others. Before I interact with those who frustrate me, G-d helps me ask, "How may I uplift your spirit today?" Now, instead of reliving the predominant portion of my life of drowning in narcissistic judgments and manipulation, EMDR gave me an effective set of tools to build back the strengths I lost over the years. I've packed my bad experiences away in containers to deal with later instead of at two in the morning. I have safe places in my mind to go to so I can remember all the blessings that I have in my life. I strive to serve others and know that they depend on me. And, I have allies.

My therapist helped me stop ruminating and evict all the narcissists. When I feel like the little kid on the porch, I've learned to love my child self by going to Bam, my new mother figure. When six-year-old me faces challenging things and needs someone to lean on, my relationship with Bam strengthens the feelings of unconditional love with which she filled my heart.

I remember the time when my brother and I were playing with our food. Instead of getting in trouble, Bam made mashed potatoes for the next meal. She then picked up some of them with her hands, made a snowball, and then showed us how to suck them out of our hands through a circle she made with her thumb and index finger. We got to have fun and figure out many ways to eat those mashed potatoes through our fingers! This experience stayed with me so strongly that I taught my kids the same game. When the teenager in me struggles, Dr. Hoffman from high school comes to mind. He felt excitement for the good things that I did and saw unlimited potential in me.

All these things led me to reinvent myself with new clothes, new glasses, and a new signature, all of which remind me of my newly found confidence. I now understand that I do not need to seek the approval of others. Only G-d can validate me, and He is perfect. I have containers all over the place. My safe place is on the beach with Laura in the Florida Keys, soaking in the sun's rays, smelling the salt water, and listening to the waves gently roll up onto my toes in the sand. With G-d behind me, Laura at my side, Bam's unconditional love, and Dr. Hoffman's excitement for my unlimited potential, I can do anything and face anyone. I am grateful to Him because I no longer carry such a heavy load.

ABOUT the AUTHOR

Steve Schechter is a Jewish educator, writer, and speaker dedicated to helping disengaged or spiritually curious Jews rediscover meaning in *shul* life and Jewish prayer. Drawing on years of personal reflection and community engagement, Steve approaches the question of *why go to shul?* with warmth, clarity, and an understanding of the barriers that keep people away.

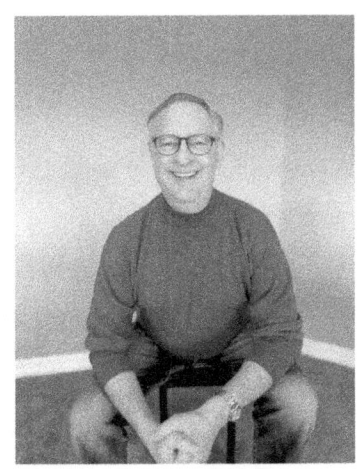

Steve has led adult education workshops, facilitated informal learning sessions, and developed resources that make Jewish ritual and liturgy accessible to modern audiences.

Steve lives in Longmont, Colorado, with his wife, Laura. He finds spiritual grounding in both traditional prayer and honest questioning.

steve.schechter@inkandinsight.us

Social Links:
Facebook: facebook.com/steve.schechter.58
LinkedIn: linkedin.com/in/steveschechteredu/
Instagram: @avra6
linktr.ee: @steve.schechter6
Threads: @avra6
X: @shamarllc
Fiverr: @steveschecht426

Chapter 12

Dichotomy

Marc Longwith

The year I turned 20 was the year everything broke.

My sister, her husband, and their daughter, my goddaughter, were killed in a head-on collision. Two weeks later, I suffered an almost-fatal gunshot wound. The bullet tore through all three arteries in my leg. Five hours in surgery. I almost died and nearly lost my leg.

Three months after that, I caught my girlfriend of six years cheating. I didn't just lose the love of my life; I lost the dream I'd wrapped my future around. A dream I had confused with safety. With wholeness.

Grieving that dream took me four years. Those four years were some of the wildest experiences of my life, led by drugs, alcohol, and emotional confusion.

Then Came 2024

Different storm, same weight, only this time I didn't have the naivety of youth to soften the blow. I had the full self-awareness of a 45-year-old man.

My business partner and I split. I had to rebuild from nothing. The woman I loved deeply, the one I poured my entire soul into and invested every ounce of who I am, the one I thought would ride or die with me, left as soon as life got hard.

My father died on Christmas Day. And I was stuck between Colombia and the States, feeling more lost, more uprooted, more alone than ever.

But Here's What All of it Taught Me:

> *The truth lives in the middle.*
> *The richness of life is in the contradiction.*
> *You can hold grief and gratitude in the same breath. You can feel broken and blessed at the same time.*
> *This isn't about compartmentalizing. It's about expansion.*
> *It's about making room to carry the weight of both joy and suffering, and becoming strong enough to stand in both.*
> *I playfully state that everything is a dichotomy, and honestly, it is. Yet the spectrum in between is the dance we must learn to master.*

Here are three of my top examples:

1. The longest mile between the head & the heart
2. Masculine & feminine balance
3. Productivity & fulfillment

Before we get started, let's get naked.
Because the truth is, you can't heal when you hide.
The shadow doesn't dissolve just by being seen; it demands to be integrated.
So, if we're going to do this work, let's be clear: this isn't surface-level.
It's all or nothing.
Others can afford to play it safe. I can't.
When it comes to *me*, there's no half-in, no pretending.

I have to strip it all back.

No masks. No branding. No carefully curated bullshit.

Just what's real. What hurts. What haunts. What I'm still ashamed to admit.

Because that's where the freedom lives.

I'll go first, of course.

Because leadership doesn't start with answers.

It starts with honesty.

I remember 20-year-old me sitting outside the apartment of the man my girlfriend was cheating on me with. Glock 27 .40 caliber, in hand. The same gun. The same caliber that nearly ended my life three months earlier.

My heart was racing. I could see them through the window: him, his friends, and her. Laughing. Relaxed. Happy. Like, none of it meant anything.

And I felt it. That fire in the bones. My stare was locked, pupils burning with pure, unfiltered rage.

I had one goal.

Kill every motherfucker in that room. Then turn the gun on myself and end it, *for good*.

But then something shifted.

Like a movie scene, dim light by the door, the camera panning out above me, like there was a spotlight on my soul.

And I heard it. A voice. A presence. Not from outside, but from somewhere deeper.

"Marc... what the fuck are you doing, man?"

I remember answering, "What the fuck does it look like?"

"You really want to throw your life away?"

"What fucking life?" I spoke.

That's when it hit me.

I was *meant* for more than this.

More than revenge. More than pain. More than ending it all just to make a point.

And somehow, I found the strength to walk away.

Let me be clear; *walking away took more courage than going in guns blazing*.

I grew up around violence. Walking away always felt weak. But this time?

This time, it was a different kind of fight.

A battle with myself.

Over time, the noise settled.

The head and the heart found each other again.

And I felt something I hadn't in a long time: *relief*.

Like a pressure valve releasing. Like I could finally breathe.

I cried the whole way home.

That night marked the beginning of a healing journey that was anything but linear.

It took me four years to fully grieve her, to stop imagining a life built around her, to stop picturing our children with her eyes, her smile, her curly hair.

It was grief not just for her, but for the dream I lost, a future I was building with someone who had already begun walking away. The same kind of grief I felt again in 2024, losing a dream that unraveled in almost the exact same way.

I'm sharing this because I want you to understand just how dark we can go as humans, and how even the brightest light is just a different angle of the same darkness.

We think light and dark are opposites. But they're not.

They're two sides of the same thing.

It's the illusion of separation that confuses us.

We keep trying to label one "good" and the other "bad," but that's not how it works.

The dark *is* the light.

The light *is* the dark.

We say life is a dance between the two, but the truth is, most of us are fighting.

Fighting the dark. Clinging to the light.

Because we've never learned how to *move* in the in-between.

The truth?

It's always in the middle.

But the only way I've ever found the middle was by swinging the damn pendulum with everything I had.

From one extreme to the other.

Like a rabid gorilla tearing through heaven and hell, refusing to stop until something clicked.

All my might.

All my energy.

All in.

I was cursed and blessed with the depth of feeling. It has been my greatest cross to bear, and my most incredible asset.

I've always been able to see things other people can't.

That gift has shown up most powerfully in the way I see *into* people, not just their stories, but their *souls*.

And because of that, I've been able to mirror back to them the parts they can't, or won't, face.

What I want to show you in this chapter is simple:

You are, by all means, completely fucked up and completely perfect, at the same time.

Nothing you ever do will *make* you feel good enough.

Not the guilt. Not the giving. Not the striving.

None of it works.

The whole point?

Acceptance

> *Radical, honest, all-of-you acceptance.*
> *Not just the polished pieces the world applauds, but the shame,*
>   *the fear, the parts you hide when no one's watching.*
> *Because here's the truth:*
> *We're all scared little boys and girls running around in adult*
>   *bodies, pretending we've got it figured out.*
> *We don't.*
> *And the biggest joke of all? We act like we've got time, like death*
>   *isn't coming sooner than we think.*

> *Life isn't meant to be solved. It's meant to be lived.*
> *Fully. Messily. Honestly.*
> *And I say that as the most fearful, controlling, anxious little boy*
> > *I've ever had the absolute pleasure of finally meeting.*
> *He's still in here.*
> *But now, I love him.*

So, as you read this, I want you to remember one thing:

Your Vote Counts the Most

> *Not theirs. Not mine. Not the world's.*
> *Love yourself, radically.*
> *Let yourself be the beautiful mess that you are.*
> *Because in the end, you won't remember the likes, the applause,*
> > *or the approval.*
> *You'll remember the experiences that molded you.*
> *The ones that broke you open.*
> *And the ones that finally made you whole.*

The Longest Mile: From the Head to the Heart

My mother wasn't the picture of perfect parenting, but she did have wisdom.

And the line that stuck with me most was this:

"The longest mile is from the head to the heart."

That line was profound and cracked something open in me.

Because the truth is, our hearts often don't catch up with our minds for years.

You can *know* something logically, but *feel* the opposite for a long damn time.

And understanding that truth has been the difference between shame and grace in my own healing.

It's like joining a jiu jitsu gym and learning all the theory in the first month, moves, leverage, strategy, but not being able to pull off a single one for the next ten years.

That's a real mindfuck.

But it taught me something:

I have to give myself grace while my heart catches up.

Grace for the parts of me still learning to let go.

Still grieving. Still adjusting. Still becoming.

Most of life is tangible; we train, we measure, we fix.

But the inner world? That world doesn't follow any linear path.

In that world, healing moves like water, not a checklist.

And I've had to learn to *allow* the current to carry me—even when it's not comfortable.

One of the biggest shifts in my journey has been this:

Learning to Hold Space for Two Truths at Once

As men, we compartmentalize.

We label. We box. We try to keep shit clean and linear.

But emotions don't operate like that.

We were never taught how to *feel*, let alone *feel multiple things at once*.

So we default to suppression, because feeling everything at the same time?

It feels like weakness.

But that's the lie.

The real weakness is pretending we're fine while bottling everything up.

Because what we suppress doesn't die, it festers.

It clogs the system.

Like cutting off an electrical current or blocking a river. Eventually, it blows.

And that explosion?

It shows up as disease, rage, shame, confusion, sometimes all at once.

This lesson became real for me—*again*—in 2025.

In the wreckage left behind after the death of my father and the end of a relationship with a woman I fully intended to spend my life with.

A woman I built my future around.

A woman I gave *everything* to.

I loved her with the kind of depth that rewrites your DNA.

I shaped my days, my dreams, my direction, my vision, around us.

And yet—

I had to hold the memory of what we had with love and tenderness *while* facing the truth in the same breath—

That she couldn't meet me where I was going.

That she wasn't ready.

And I couldn't carry both of us anymore.

I wanted it to work more than I've ever wanted anything in my life.

But I was tired.

Tired of being abandoned while in the relationship.

And even more so, completely betrayed in the end.

Nothing burns more than the broken promises of the woman you love!

That shit is confusing.

To feel so much love for someone and still know you have to let them go?

That's *work*.

And it requires the ability to sit in multiple layers of truth without losing yourself.

Maybe that's why women are better at multitasking; they don't need to stuff everything into separate boxes to make sense of it.

The point is this:

The longest mile can be shortened if you learn to *feel and process in real time.*

That's a skill most men are missing. And it's raw, I won't lie.

It looks like waking up in tears because your chest is crushed by grief,

and still getting up, putting on some Goggins, and hitting the gym like a warrior.

Then—

On your way out of the gym, sweat still clinging to your skin like the grief that hasn't fully left your body, you bump into her.

The very source of your heartbreak.

The ghost you've been trying to make peace with.

Alive. Right in front of you.

And she's not alone.

She's with him.

The new guy she moved on to within a week.

Like plug and play—

As if everything you shared was just a warm-up for her next chapter.

And now you've got to access something deeper than muscle:

Maturity.

Presence.

Self-control.

Not the kind you fake to seem "unbothered."

But the kind that says:

I've grieved you. I've forgiven you. And I've chosen myself.

Even if your heart skips.

Even if part of you still aches.

Even if your nervous system lights up with memory.

This is the test.

Can you *stay sovereign* in the presence of what once shattered you?

That's not weakness.

That's not confusion.

That's *integration*.

And it takes *work*.

It takes practice. Awareness. Breath. Reflection.

Otherwise, we stay trapped in a loop, operating from the lowest version of ourselves because we don't know how to hold everything at once.

My goal in this chapter is to give you a process.

A way to *move through* your emotions without drowning in them.

To shorten the mile from head to heart.

Because we don't know how much time we really have, and I, for one, don't want to waste it.

But I also don't want to destroy my future because I never resolved my past.

So, Here's the Truth:

If you don't feel it now, you'll carry it later.

And it'll cost you more than you can imagine.

We think we're doing ourselves a favor by pushing through.

But all we're doing is *delaying the detonation.*

It's like Algebra.

Miss the fundamentals in semester one, and you're screwed for the rest of the year.

You'll keep trying to solve problems with a broken equation.

And then you wake up at 40 wondering why your life looks more like a hallucination than the reality you actually wanted.

"The Integration Chair" Exercise

Here is an exercise to help you shorten the longest mile, from the head to the heart.

Purpose:

To bridge the gap between intellectual understanding and emotional embodiment by confronting a truth you know in your mind but haven't yet felt in your heart.

Instructions:

1. **Get two chairs.**
   - Place them facing each other in a quiet room. One is for your *head* (logic), the other for your *heart* (emotion).
2. **Sit in the *head* Chair.**
   - Speak out loud, as your rational mind. Say the truth you've known for a while.
   - Examples: *She wasn't good for me.*

- *He did the best he could.*
- *It's over.*
- Speak from intellect. Detached. Clinical. Straight facts.
3. **Now switch.**
    - Sit in the *heart* chair.
    - Let yourself feel everything that contradicts what your mind just said.
    - Say it raw, emotional, broken.
    - *But I still love her.*
    - *It wasn't enough.*
    - *Why didn't they fight for me?*
    - Let your voice tremble. Let tears come. Let anger rise.
4. **Repeat the dialogue.**
    - Go back and forth as many rounds as needed until something *clicks*.
    - The moment where both voices soften. When you can sit in either chair and say: *Both are true.*
    - That's when you have walked the mile.
5. **Close with these questions. (Write it down.)**
    - *Now that I've made space for both truths, what can I let go of?*
    - *What can I carry with grace?"*

Why This Exercise Works:

You can't logically process your way through grief. But you also can't let emotion run wild forever. This exercise creates a felt experience of integration—head and heart no longer enemies, but allies.

The Sacred Dance: Balancing Masculine and Feminine

The interplay between masculine and feminine energy is one of my favorite subjects because it's how we fully engage with life.

We live in a world obsessed with extremes. Polarization is now a marketing strategy. Pick a side. Get clicks. Stir the pot. But real life–

the rich, meaningful kind–exists in the dance between energies, not in their division.

Jordan Peterson once said, "You should be a monster, an absolute threat, and then learn how to control it."

I agree. I've spent most of my life becoming that threat. I've forged myself into a weapon; physically, mentally, emotionally. But what makes that power sacred is restraint. Discipline. Direction. Love.

Masculine

I learned to fight as a boy and eventually stepped into the cage as a professional MMA fighter. I've trained with elite operators, learned to shoot, to track, to anticipate movement and energy in a room before a word is spoken. My stepfather, along with much of my family, was a criminal. That reality shaped me. It gave me an instinct for danger and a deep understanding of what it means to protect.

This isn't the "divine masculine." But let's not confuse sentiment with softness. At its core, masculinity is *presence*. Protection. Direction. If I'm to protect myself and those I love from the enemy, I must understand the enemy. Think like him, feel like him, and be prepared to dismantle him completely if needed.

That's the edge I carry. But being a man isn't just about shooting a Glock, growing a beard, or throwing hands. While my future sons will know those skills, because I believe competence breeds confidence, that's only one side of the equation.

Feminine

Here's the part most men won't admit: I am by far one of the most feminine men I know. I love to cuddle, I love to nest and craft my home, I love to dote on my partner, I love to nurture those that I love, and honestly, people in general.

I have learned to listen and receive rather than to speak and guide all the time.

I think we must learn to dance between the two extremes and to realize they're not a box but an interplay.

In a world that wants us to be so rigid, I implore you to find a sacred balance, a blend, a place in the middle.

We can protect our daughters and our wives viciously and still hold safe spaces for them to soften and find a home in.

We can stand tall and strong, and build life brick by brick, and still fall into the arms of our lovers, sob deeply, and release the pressure that the world places on our shoulders.

We are so much more than we give ourselves not only credit for, but the permission to be.

We are not boxes, we are not forgotten, we are the cornerstone of this world, and we carry the weight of it on our shoulders so heavily that our backs almost feel like they could break at any moment. Still, every morning, we rise up and stand tall, and often even pretend we are doing just fine. So we can protect the ones we love, the places we've built, and the image we've crafted for ourselves as the strong ones.

I commend you, I really do, and I also implore you to allow yourself to drop deeply into the softest sides of yourselves and to give yourself the grace and the love that you not only deserve but you need.

To coddle that little boy inside of you that had to grow up so fucking early. It was so unfair for him to have to carry the weight of a man as a boy. To have to stand tall and suck it up and not show any emotion. To be praised for his stoicism when he was just a boy who was scared and wanted nothing more than to be protected by his mommy and daddy.

The weight we carry as men is unbearable at times, and for me, I know that the world rests on my shoulders. I don't think that will ever change, I don't think I will ever not desire to serve and to carry the burden for others. That is just who I am and how I am built. It is my honor to hold the line and carry the weight. Yet, as men, we need respect and validation. We need to be recognized for the load we so valiantly choose to carry for the world and the ones we love.

So right now, I want to give you permission. Permission for two things. To find a safe space to set the weight down (don't worry, you can pick it back up), and to find the kindness, the love, and the compassion to gently care for that little boy who has been built upon a repetitive cycle of protection and fear.

Like Russian nesting dolls, one on top of the other. Protecting the smaller one until you became so strong and so powerful that you were able to gather all of those little boys up and hold them in your arms and protect each and every one of them. The 3-year-old version of you, the eight-year-old version, the 12-year-old version, and so on.

This is where we must learn to drop deeply into our feminine, nurturing, and loving side of ourselves and to unapologetically hold space for each version of us that was never protected, never truly seen, and never loved properly.

Only then can we heal the divine masculine within us and show up powerfully for those who need us to do for them what we never did for ourselves.

You see, that is our job, that is our mission, to break the cycle, to destroy the line. To develop such deep awareness that we are operating proactively in our lives and not creating another generation of fucked up children who lack the love, the skills, and the capacity to function as whole adults and not adult children.

I like to say that we are all little boys and girls running around in adult bodies. Let's normalize the opposite. Let's create a generation of emotionally mature, strong and soft adults who have the skills and the hearts to pour themselves into this world and the generations that come after us, so we can leave this world a better place than we found it and have our work echo for eternity.

Productivity & Fulfillment

Let's bring this back to real life.

This is where it counts. Where dreams are either lived or buried. And let's be honest, most of us beat the living fuck out of ourselves in the process.

This section is your practical guide. The *how*. The blueprint for achieving machine-like productivity *without* sacrificing your soul. How to build, create, dominate, and still enjoy the wild ride.

And when I say *destination*, I mean death.

That's where we're all headed, and you should be ready for it at any moment.

I learned this early. Growing up around high-level violence. Training with special operators. Being shaped, molded, really, by legitimate psychopaths. Some by blood. Some by choice. I've seen what it looks like to master destruction. And I've seen what it takes to channel that power into purpose.

If you understood the level of emotional control I hold in contrast to my capacity for violence, you'd understand why I say I'm proud of who I've become.

Because despite the darkness I've been steeped in, all I want now is to give love to this world.

That's the dichotomy. The razor's edge.

It's the entire fucking point.

But I digress, back to what matters in the day-to-day.

Here's the Truth:

Fulfillment and productivity are not the same thing.

Most men chase productivity, hoping it will deliver fulfillment. But that's a false metric.

We are *human beings*, not *human doings*.

That phrase landed hard when I first heard it from a client named Al. I remember thinking, *Damn. That's it. That's the entire sermon right there.*

We're measuring the right longing with the wrong metric.

It's like that old country song, "Looking for love in all the wrong places..."

Or the time I was venting to my friend Rebecca about the lack of support I felt from a partner, and she said:

"Marc, you can't get milk from the hardware store."

So let me say it straight:
Productivity is not fulfillment.
I'll say it again:
Productivity is not fulfillment.

The paradox of high performers, especially men, is this myth: *The more you accomplish, the happier you'll be.*

But in reality? The more you accomplish, the *emptier* you may feel. Why?

Because you're shopping for soul in a store that only sells status.

Let's go deeper, neurologically.

Every time you chase a goal, your brain releases dopamine. The pursuit is the high. The grind lights you up. But the second you arrive, you crash.

Because your brain is wired for survival, *not* satisfaction.

It rewards the *chase*, not the *completion*.

So, what do you do? You move the goalpost. You create a new target. Another hit. Another climb.

And you wonder why you never feel like you've *arrived*.

That's the illusion of success.

It's not just in your mind, it's in your wiring.

And the system *loves* it.

Our entire economy thrives on keeping you chasing the next hit.

You've been conditioned like a lab rat pressing the lever, hoping *this time* the reward will satisfy.

But it never does.

So, what's the real answer?

Service. Contribution. Giving Back.

Fulfillment isn't found in the next achievement. It's found in *meaning*.

In helping others.

In using your pain as fuel to make life better for someone else.

That's where the peace is. That's where the soul exhales.

So, here's my final question:

How Will You Give Back?

How will you make your mark on this world?

What is your unique genius, and how will you share it in a way that *aligns* with your soul and *impacts* the people who need you most?

That's your real work.

Not just to *do more*, but to *be more*.

Not just to build, but to *be built*.

And maybe, just maybe, to die fulfilled.

ABOUT the AUTHOR

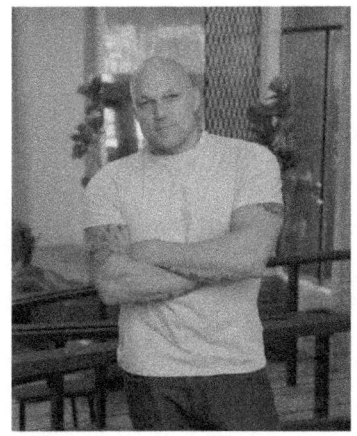

Marc Anthony Longwith is a transformational advisor, speaker, and founder of Evolved Entrepreneur, a movement helping high-level professionals break through internal limitations and realign with their true power. With a background that spans elite hospitality leadership, professional martial arts, and building a seven-figure coaching business, Marc blends grit, emotional intelligence, and spiritual insight to guide clients through profound reinvention. Known for his raw honesty, strategic brilliance, and deep empathy, he works with executives, athletes, U.S. military special operators, and mission-driven creators ready to evolve beyond success into significance. Whether on stage, in private advisory sessions, or through his signature programs, Marc teaches leaders how to rewire their identity, master emotional resilience, and step fully into their purpose. He is a trusted guide for those navigating transitions and seeking to create a legacy from authenticity. His work is not about surface-level motivation—it's about rewiring the soul to lead from depth, conviction, and unshakable clarity.

Chapter 13

MENifest

A Love Greater Than Fear
Dr. Vincent Johnson Jr.

It was around 11:30 on Easter night, 1972, when I was awakened by a strange sound coming from the living room of our small two-bedroom house in Denver, Colorado. The air was thick with the smell of alcohol and cigarette butts, but even at five years old, I was already used to that.

What I wasn't used to was *this* sound. I heard a man singing along with his guitar, matching the guitar notes exactly. Later in life, I would come to understand this as *scat soloing*. Curious, I climbed out of bed and snuck quietly around the corner into the living room. It was easy. Both my parents were passed out drunk. In my neighborhood, we didn't call it *intoxicated*—we called it *polluted*, or in Ebonics, *pie-looted*, or *tore up from the floor up*.

Weekends in our home were wild, filled with card games, loud laughter, drinking, cursing, and the inevitable argument. Then came the calm after the storm, when Mom and my stepdad were passed out cold. But this sound, this *amazing* sound, pulled me in like a magnet. It was as if I were floating, carried straight into the front room by some invisible current.

To my surprise, the sound was coming from The Merv Griffin Show, one of the most popular late-night talk shows on TV at the time. Every now and then, I'd get to stay up late and catch a glimpse of TV, mostly because my parents' drinking habits left them unaware. When Merv Griffin came on, you knew it was the last show of the night. After that, just static.

If I had been caught watching TV, there would've been hell to pay. But I was too taken by the music to care. The emotional pull it had on me was overwhelming. I was caught in a field of emotional frequency I didn't have words for yet. It was as if each note tapped into a different emotional color. So, I hurried to the floor in front of the TV.

On the screen was a man who looked like he could've been one of my uncles, playing guitar and singing at the same time. This, to the best of my memory, was the first time I experienced something that would follow me for the rest of my life: *synesthesia*. Synesthesia is the phenomenon where the senses cross wires, when a sound is so beautiful, it causes a physical or emotional reaction. Goosebumps. A smile. Even tears. In my case, it was wide-eyed wonder and total surrender. My senses had been hijacked, and I loved it. That was the moment I knew what I wanted to do with my life. I wanted to make people feel *this*. That night marked the beginning of my lifelong journey and the discovery of what would become my personal method of self-soothing.

The man on the screen was none other than George Benson, performing his breakthrough hit, *On Broadway*, in a way only a true master could. His control over the guitar, his ability to sing and scat simultaneously, blew my five-year-old mind. I'd never seen or heard anything like it.

When the performance ended, the TV went to static. I turned it off and scurried back to bed, hoping not to wake anyone. If I had I been caught, I would've gotten it *good*. But I made it back safe. That night, lying in bed, I drifted in and out of sleep, replaying the music in my head. I kept wondering, *How can a human being make a sound like that?* My journey had officially begun.

The next morning, my mother, as usual, walked me to school. But something was different; I was electric. Excited! I couldn't stop talking about what I had seen the night before and how it had lit something inside me. I remember looking up at her, eyes wide, as I described the man, the guitar, the feeling. Knowing that my mom would forgive my transgression of sneaking out of my bed so late at night, and possibly a little guilt for not being *Parent of the Year*, she looked down, smiled, and said, "Baby, we can't afford a guitar right now, but I think they're giving violin lessons at your school."

I thought to myself, *Well, if I can't get a guitar, maybe I can get a violin and still be cool like George Benson.* I didn't know it yet, but that violin would be one of my first lessons in how to survive the hood. You see, where I grew up, playing an instrument was seen as soft. *Sissy*, they called it. Football, wrestling, or karate were the cool things to do at that age. And I wasn't a big kid, not by any stretch, which made things harder. Add in the intense anxiety I already carried from home, and you can imagine how quickly playing the violin would turn into an internal and external battlefield.

My home life? Let's just say it was soaked in dysfunction. Today, they'd call it trauma and abuse, severe trauma, honestly, mixed with neglect and abandonment. But back then, we just called it *a rough road*.

My stepfather was a hard-working man, but he had demons. And, like in so many families, his issues spilled out into everything, especially our relationship. Or really, the absence of one.

I carried anxiety like it was stitched into my skin. I was named after my biological father, "Big Vince"—so naturally, I was "Little Vince." And every time my stepfather called my name, I felt it in my gut. There was always a sharpness to his voice. Aggression. And almost always, it came with a curse word.

Vincent! I told you to wash the dishes! Dammit, boy, what the hell is wrong with you?

The sound of my name coming from his mouth hit like lightning striking a tree. My nervous system would go haywire, fight, flight, fawn, or freeze. For me, it was *freeze*. I'd stutter, too terrified to speak clearly. It got so bad that my mom eventually took me to a therapist. After a few sessions, the therapist made it clear: the issue wasn't me, it was my stepfather.

Still, my mom, curious and creative as always, tried to give me what she could. She looked into instruments, and sure enough, she signed me up for violin at school.

I remember that first day in violin class like it was yesterday. I was buzzing with excitement. I was finally going to get my very own instrument. Our teacher called our names one by one, handing out violins like sacred treasures.

Before we even drew a bow, she gave us a serious warning: "Take care of this instrument and guard it with your life."

We took her words to heart. This wasn't just a school supply, it was a key to something greater. She gave us our first lesson, but bless her heart, it only lasted about 15 minutes. That's all her ears could take. It must've sounded like a dozen cats being strangled. My hands ached from the strings, my neck cramped up, and I swore my ears were bleeding from the awful noises I was making, but I was smiling. Because that sound, as awful as it was, was *mine*. It was the start of something.

When the bell rang, I packed up my violin like it was a trophy and practically floated out of the classroom. This was the '70s, so walking home from school was normal. We traveled in packs for safety, but I had no idea the pack I was walking with would turn on me.

The teasing began almost immediately: *Vincent plays a violin! Only sissies play violins!*

They laughed, pointed, and pushed. I was small, sure, but I was also full of rage. A rage born from the chaos at home. And, being sensitive by nature, that teasing hit harder than any punch. But I wasn't about to take abuse outside the house, too. Not anymore. That's when I learned how to fight.

Almost every day after school, I had to scrap my way home. For weeks. Eventually, a neighbor told my mom what was happening. She made the tough decision to return the violin. And just like that, it was gone. But what I lost in strings, I gained in fists. My fighting skills skyrocketed.

Not long after, I got my next instrument: a Mickey Mouse drum set. My mom helped me set it up right there in my room. She closed the door and let me go wild. It was magical, for a moment. But then my stepfather came home.

Put that God_m boy outside with them d—m drums, I don't wanna hear all that shit!

And believe it or not, *that* was him being nice. So there I was, out in the front yard with my tiny drum set, banging away while the neighbors stared. The drums didn't last long. I came home one day and, poof, they were gone. No explanation. No warning. Just silence where there used to be rhythm.

A few years later, we moved to Park Hill, another part of Denver. Locals called it *Hillside Park or BoardWalk*. It was more integrated than the neighborhood we'd come from. And, while that might sound like a good thing, it came with new challenges. Back in my old school, I was ahead of the curve. In Park Hill, I found myself behind. These kids, mostly white, were more advanced in English and math.

After placement testing, I was put in a lower English class. It hit me like a brick. *Maybe my stepfather was right, I thought. Maybe I am stupid.* He told me that often enough, why wouldn't I believe it? *You dumb little motherf—er!*

Boy, you ain't never gon' be nothin, you're digressing instead of progressing! That became my internal dialogue. A broken record I couldn't turn off, even when the music played. Still, I showed up. I took the hits, verbally at home, emotionally at school, and I kept going. Because what else was there to do? It was around this time that I discovered something that would change everything: I could sing. I mean, *really sing*. It felt like stumbling on a buried treasure inside myself. I had no idea it was there, just waiting.

My first big break came when Barry Manilow came to town. They were putting together a children's choir for his song, *"One Light."* And guess who got picked? Me.

Just one light, singing in the darkness...

That lyric hit me deep. It *was* me. I *was* that one light. From that moment on, I sang everywhere I went. At school, in the mirror, on the walk home. Music wasn't just my passion, it was my lifeline, my identity.

I still remember the sound of my stepfather's car pulling into the driveway each evening. I could tell just by the way he parked whether he'd been drinking. If he had, oddly enough, it was a relief. A drunk stepdad was better than a sober, angry one. Drunk, he didn't yell. He didn't have the energy. Being ignored became its own kind of peace.

He wasn't abusive toward my mom, Oh no! She was a fighter. But me? I took the hits. And while they weren't physical, the emotional and psychological abuse left bruises you couldn't see. I used to say, *At least he never hit me.*

I remember my mother telling my girlfriend one day, "Well, at least he made it out alive." Wow! As if that was worth some coveted blue ribbon. But as I grew older, I realized those invisible wounds ran just as deep—maybe deeper–than physical abuse. They don't fade like black eyes. They don't scab over. They linger. For years. Decades. Sometimes forever.

Eventually, I lost count of how many times the police or fire department showed up at our house. My mom and stepdad would get drunk, throw some food on the stove, pass out, and forget about it. The house would fill with smoke, the neighbors would call 911, and we'd be running outside in pajamas, coughing and confused. It became routine. Embarrassing. Humiliating. Traumatizing. I didn't know it back then, but that kind of public chaos plants seeds of anxiety deep in a kid's soul. Curtains had to be cleaned constantly.

I still hate the smell of anything burning. That smell brings it all back. But in the middle of all that madness, there were still moments of light.

One of those moments came when I got to middle school. Out of nowhere, my mom surprised me; she bought me an acoustic guitar. My first real guitar. I was shocked. Overwhelmed. Ecstatic. That gift changed everything. I went straight to the basement to play. Then I played for hours every night. I didn't know how to read music, so I just listened to records and tried to mimic what I heard.

"Greensleeves" was one of the first songs I taught myself. Then came my obsession with the folk songwriter John Denver. His voice, his guitar work, it all spoke to me in a language I finally understood.

By then, I had a reputation. I was known as a scrapper, a fighter. My nickname was "Pistol Grip" because I stayed ready for whatever. Nobody messed with me anymore. Playing the guitar didn't get me teased like the violin had. I could carry my instrument now, literally and metaphorically. But that edge, that toughness, was both a shield and a curse. I was mirroring what I'd seen my whole life: react first, defend always. That trauma started showing up at school, in my relationships, and in how I handled conflict. My mom, in her wisdom, put me in martial arts. She hoped it would help me manage my anger. And I agreed, but for a different reason. I wanted to protect *her*.

One summer afternoon during break, I was downstairs playing my guitar. The house was quiet. Mom was at work, and I was just vibing in the basement with my dog, enjoying that rare sense of peace. Then I heard the front door swing open. My stepfather had come home early for lunch. Every time he entered a room, I felt like the door got kicked open, even if it hadn't been. His energy hit before his body did. He stomped down the stairs in his work boots like an angry giant and flung the door open so hard it slammed into the wall.

God—it, Vincent! Didn't I tell you to do them god—n dishes and rake them leaves? What the f*** is wrong with you, you dumbass motherf***er? You won't be living here much longer! Soon as you turn 16, you're outta here!

Then he turned around and thundered back upstairs, slamming the door so hard behind him it shook the walls.

Then I cracked. Everything inside me, years of shame, pain, fear, rage, exploded.

I grabbed my guitar and smashed it against the cold basement floor. Once, twice, until it shattered into what felt like a thousand tiny pieces. Splinters flew across the room, strings twanged one final time, and then... silence.

I collapsed on the bed and cried. Not the kind of tears that roll gently down your face, these were the kind that choke you. I cried until I couldn't cry anymore.

A few hours later, my mom came home. She found the guitar in pieces. Then she walked into my room, saw me curled up, eyes swollen.

"Vincent, what happened to the guitar? Did you break it? Why?"

I couldn't even lift my head. "I don't know, Mom... I just got really mad."

With a concerned voice, she asked, "Did your dad come home?"

I nodded, *Yes*. "He came home, yelled at me again."

She didn't yell. She didn't ask for more. She just sat beside me and held me. See, my mother was loving. Raw, complicated, but loving. She would take time to explain very complex sociological constructs to me with kindness, gentleness, and patience. After all, she was a behavioral specialist.

Breaking that guitar was like breaking my own heart. But in that moment, it was the only thing I had control over. Everything else in my world, my emotions, my safety, my home, it all felt completely out of my hands. So I broke the one thing that was mine.

It wasn't until years later that I fully understood why my mother stayed. She was afraid, afraid of being alone in the world, afraid of starting over, afraid of not having enough. That fear? That's where my codependency began. You see, in life, I've learned there are really only two choices behind every decision we make: love or fear. Period.

My mom was the bridge between my stepfather and me. She tried to soften his roughness, to translate his rage into something I could survive. She was my buffer, my interpreter. She taught me how to read between the lines, how to find meaning in the silences and the slurs. In her eyes, his abuse was really just his twisted way of loving, protecting, maybe even preparing me. At least, that's what she told herself, and eventually, what I told myself too.

That's the thing about survival: you learn to make sense of the nonsense just to keep breathing. A few months later, I had saved up enough money cutting grass and raking leaves to buy myself a guitar. Mom took me to a little store called Sound Town. The moment we walked in, I was overwhelmed, not with fear, but with excitement. The walls were lined with guitars, keyboards, amps... it was like I'd stepped into another dimension. Even the staff treated me like I belonged. It didn't feel like a store. It felt like church, the instruments were the congregation, and the salesman was the pastor.

I saw a black guitar on the wall. That was it. That was *my* guitar. But I didn't have quite enough money. My mom, being who she was, smiled and covered the rest without hesitation.

The guy behind the counter asked, "You realize without an amp, you won't be able to hear it, right?"

I shrugged. "Yeah. I know. But we can't afford that yet."

"Well," he said, "I've got another option."

He pointed me to something he called a Rockman. "You plug your guitar in, put on headphones, and you can hear yourself play without disturbing anyone."

Mom looked at me. I looked at her. That was our path.

She reached back into her purse. Probably a bill didn't get paid that month, but I walked out of that store with a guitar, a Rockman, and a fire inside me.

From that day forward, the basement became my sanctuary. I'd spend hours down there with my headphones on, lost in sound, learning, failing, trying again. I didn't have formal training, didn't know how to read music, but my ears were my teachers. I played until my fingers ached, chasing the feelings I first had when I saw George Benson on that screen. And oh yeah, PRINCE!

I was the first in my neighborhood to learn how to play "When Doves Cry." Rather fitting for my home life. While chaos still reigned upstairs, I found peace in the strings. When my mom and stepdad argued, I'd crank the volume. When the shouting turned into slamming, I'd close my eyes and play harder.

My stepfather would occasionally come down, peek in the door, shake his head in disapproval, and walk away. Slam. Always the slam. But in that basement, I was free. Playing guitar became more than a hobby; it was therapy. It was how I learned to self-soothe. And I needed it more than ever.

After years of verbal abuse and emotional chaos, I grew numb. I was so used to being called names, so used to being dismissed, ignored, emasculated, that I started to expect it. On the rare days when things were calm, I'd get anxious. I didn't know what to do with peace. I didn't know how to relax. Fun came with guilt. Laughter was a red flag. Even joy became a trigger.

Some days I'd be hanging out with my friends, laughing and feeling like a normal kid, and then it would hit me: I had to go home. Back to the nightmare. Back to walking on eggshells. Back to holding my breath. It got so bad that my best buddy, now, Dr. Jones, like in Raiders of the Lost Ark, would have to wait until my migraines subsided in order to go have fun. But he was my patient friend, and still is to this day.

Eventually, the chaos at home all came to a head. My stepfather had been reminding me since I was a kid that I had to leave when I turned 16. *You're gone*, he'd say, *as soon as you're old enough*. But I was only 14 when the threats turned physical.

One afternoon, he came home from work early, while my mom was out. I was in the basement, playing guitar, my dog Smoky at my feet, minding my business, safe, for a moment. But then I heard him coming down the stairs like a storm in boots. He burst in, angry, hammer in hand. He raised that hammer just inches from my face, his eyes full of something darker than anger, hatred. I stood frozen, silent, my soul detached from my body. I had never felt that type of hate from any human up until that point. But love doesn't feel like that, and it sure as hell doesn't sound like that.

It would be many years before I understood the full weight of the trauma I endured. Still, I internalized the message. I began to believe that if I just endured enough, if I just loved enough, I could make the pain stop. That maybe I could love someone into wholeness.

I didn't yet realize that love without safety is not love. It's survival. It was then that I began asking family members if I could stay with them, hoping someone would say yes. Most of them said, *No, Vincent. You need to stay home. You have to protect your mom.* Hadn't I been doing that my whole life? From the age of two until then, I had been shielding her. But who was shielding me? She married him. She chose him. And that's when the shift happened.

I asked my grandmother, my dad's mom, Nana. And to my surprise, she said yes. She wanted me. I remember the moment I told my stepfather I was leaving. He laughed. He said my dad, my Nana, and everyone on that side of the family didn't love me. But I thought to myself, *How much worse could it be?* If this was his version of love, I was willing to take my chances.

Moving in with Nana changed everything. She lived just a few blocks away, but stepping into her home felt like entering another world. There was calm. There was structure. There was love. She had a piano upstairs that I'd play for hours, practicing the same chords over and over until I got them right. Not once did she complain. In fact, she'd sit there clapping after every little tune, like she was front row at Carnegie Hall. She gave me something I hadn't had in a long time: a sense of being wanted.

Those two years I spent with her during high school were lifesaving. Literally. What I didn't know then was that healing was already underway. Little did I know, a year after moving in, I'd be playing with the Denver Symphony Orchestra, and hearing that same kind of applause, only louder. Although Nana didn't play piano herself, there were a few gifted musicians on my mother's side of the family. One of them was my Aunt Judy. Now *she* was a firecracker.

Aunt Judy was the first Black woman to own an appraisal business in Colorado. She took after my Uncle Jesse Johnson, who ran the first Black-owned real estate and mortgage company in the state. These weren't just family members; they were pioneers. And Aunt Judy? Man, she didn't take no mess from anybody. She'd tell you off with a smile and a raised eyebrow, then sit down and play the blues like she was born in the Mississippi Delta. She taught me my first blues riff. Showed me once. I never forgot it.

On both sides of my family, there were protectors. My maternal grandparents, Maxine and Leo Hood, showed me what real love looked like. Their home became a refuge as well. Just three blocks from the chaos of my mother's house, I'd walk over any time, day or night, and find peace. Sometimes I'd climb into bed between the two of them and watch late-night religious shows while eating cereal straight out of the box. It wasn't fancy, but it was safe.

My grandfather, Leo, was a railroad chef and a master with a blade.

He taught me how to sharpen knives, plant a real garden, and cook Thanksgiving dinner from scratch. I still remember the rhythm of his sharpening steel, like he was playing hambone on a washboard and slapping his knee. There was music in everything that man did. Even the way he sliced turkey. Those were sacred memories, the kind that stay stitched into your soul. And I held onto them. Still do.

On Friday nights, the whole family would gather at my grandparents' house. The adults played cards, drank a little, and talked smack, while the kids sat in front of the TV watching *Sanford and Son*, *Archie Bunker*, and our favorite, *Good Times*. We laughed. We ate. We belonged. *That*, that was love. And I would spend the rest of my life chasing that feeling.

By 14, I was living with Nana, spending most of my time down in the basement surrounded by music. That's where I learned to play multiple instruments. I had no fancy setup, no teachers, just the drive to create something beautiful out of my pain. That basement became my sanctuary.

One day, sitting with my guitar and at my buddy's house, Dr. Jones, I looked over at my boys—weed smoke hanging in the air—and said, "My guitar's gonna take me around the world."

They laughed. I didn't blame them. It sounded crazy, and to be honest, I laughed too. But deep down, I knew. I could feel it. Just two months later, that "crazy" turned into a plane ticket. I got accepted into *Up With People*, a global youth performance group that used music to inspire change. And just like that, I was gone. From Denver basements to world stages. It happened fast. But trauma doesn't need a passport; it packed itself and went right along with me.

The years of emotional and mental abuse would continue to show up in my life, replaying like a scratched record. I didn't see it at first. I just thought I was choosing the wrong relationships, trusting the wrong people. But I was reenacting the only script I'd ever known, codependency, silence in the face of dysfunction, hoping love could fix what fear created.

But it wasn't all bad. That pain gave me armor, emotional calluses that would help me navigate one of the toughest industries out there.

The music business will break your heart if you're not ready, and even if you are, it will bring you to your knees. Rejection is the norm, not the exception. You can't just be talented, you've gotta be resilient. You've gotta be cracked open enough to feel, but strong enough not to fall apart. That's what synesthesia became for me, transforming trauma into tone. Feeling the pain and turning it into sound. I became an alchemist.

In the early 2000s, I was back in Denver and, just as my career was gaining traction, life threw me a curve I didn't see coming. I didn't have a place to live.

My grandmother had passed away and left me her piano. I didn't have a proper place to store the piano, so I kept it in the back of my Chevy Blazer. At night, I'd park somewhere, pull it out, and play while my wolf-dog, Shilo, would sleep in the backseat.

I had no home and was overworked, and carrying around the piano from place to place. Then, on top of all that, I lost my ability to walk. One day, I was performing in the studio, the next, I couldn't walk.

That piano became my therapy, my church, and the local crackheads and drug dealers were my audience, literally! And wouldn't you know it, while sleeping in that Blazer, unable to walk without support, I got signed to a major publishing label. Talk about divine timing. It was a blessing and a curse. I was in pain, but I was being seen. I had no money, but I had a voice. I couldn't stand, but I could write, and that's what I did. I wrote out the pain.

One song called "Would I Lie?" hit the charts, and another one, called "Mr. Lonely" was placed on TV. My group, Lyric, was just me and my singing partner, Orlando, who helped me get off the streets into a place to live. We sounded like a soulful Darryl Hall and John Oats, or Simon and Garfunkel. That season taught me the difference between chasing comfort and creating it. The world tells us to look outside ourselves, to find healing in a person, a paycheck, a pill, a pastor, or a politician. But I learned the real medicine is already inside. Music was never just a career for me; it was survival. It was my language when words failed, my compass when I lost direction, and my sanctuary when home didn't feel safe.

Doctors had their theories about why I couldn't walk, and I went in for a major surgery. I was only in my twenties, and I was terrified. But here's the thing about fear: it's a brilliant teacher. It'll introduce you to parts of yourself you never knew existed. When I couldn't walk, I had to learn how to be still. Stillness, for someone like me, was torture at first. But in that stillness, I heard a different rhythm. A quieter one.

In 2021, life turned up the volume again. I suffered severe burns, first-, second-, and third-degree, across my upper torso and arm. It was brutal. That night, I had my first, and hopefully only, near-death experience. Alone. In a hospital bed. Every breath felt like fire. But with each breath, I remembered something sacred: the name *Yahweh*. *Yah,* the inhale. *Weh*, the exhale. They say that's the first name every newborn calls on, just by breathing. And for the next four to six months, every breath I took was a reminder: I was still here. Still breathing. Still being called. I couldn't hold a guitar. I couldn't sing. I couldn't even sit upright for long without feeling like I was on fire.

So I did the only thing I knew how to do: I turned inward. I meditated. I prayed. I studied scripture, biology, sound, light, and the anatomy of the human body. That's when I began to understand something ancient, yet newly revealed to me–what happens when light, sound, and steam converge. I'd always been drawn to the idea of spiritual threes:

Mind, body, spirit.

Father, Son, Holy Spirit.

Heart, gut, mind.

That trifecta began to make more sense as I sat in stillness, healing not just my skin, but something deeper. The accident, though painful, became my classroom. I realized I hadn't just been chasing healing, I'd been chasing the chance to save someone: my mother.

Every time I let someone cross my boundaries, every time I put someone on a pedestal to my own detriment, every time I let myself be drained emotionally, I was reenacting the same pattern: trying to save the woman who never asked to be saved. That realization shook me to my core. It changed me. It showed me how to create boundaries.

In 2023, life hit me again, this time with a minor stroke. It started with bell's palsy. The entire left side of my face went numb. I couldn't smile or blink properly. I lost full function. My speech was slurred, my eye watered constantly, and food would fall out of my mouth when I tried to eat. I couldn't sing, and stepping into the recording booth felt foreign. I felt like a ghost of the artist I had once been.

While I was still dealing with bell's palsy, doctors thought I might have lung cancer after I was hospitalized with a variety of symptoms, including: multifocal pneumonia, an abscessed tooth, lockjaw, an ear infection, and a sinus infection The weight of it all was staggering.

When I was released, I walked home from the hospital. I needed to think. To breathe. To soothe myself. I talked to God with every step.

I passed a storefront window in downtown Denver and caught my reflection. I stopped and stared at my distorted face. Tears welled up. I saw a version of myself I didn't recognize, but somehow, I still knew the man staring back at me.

That was a turning point. I realized I'd allowed stress, once again, to quietly unravel me from the inside out. It was time to make a change for the sake of my health, for real this time. I couldn't sing. I could barely talk without a whistle at the end of every S or F.

Then something funny and unexpected happened. I discovered that I could rap. That's right, I embraced the whistle and leaned into it like a hip-hop LL Cool J.

I wrote and recorded a full rap album. It wasn't just music; it was medicine. My Rocky Balboa moment. And you know what? It made people laugh. It made *me* laugh, and I was truly alright with that. Even in my brokenness, I was still creating. Still reaching. Still alive.

Eventually, the paralysis faded, the swelling went down, and my face returned to normal. From time to time, I still get phantom pain, a strange reminder of the storm I survived. And every time it stings, I smile. Because that pain? That's proof I made it. After all these years of peeling back the layers, I've learned a few essential truths.

Mental and emotional abuse is like strong invisible poison; it doesn't leave bruises, but it corrodes you from within. It leaves the kind of damage that only becomes visible under a spiritual microscope, and even then, only in the dark.

One of the most powerful lessons I've learned is this: being adaptable can be a gift, but only in the right environments. At work, for instance, I can lead from the front, fall back when needed, or simply be a team player. I'm malleable. That's a strength.

But in my personal life, I've discovered that being too flexible in toxic or dysfunctional situations can be deadly. When you come from a background of trauma, you're taught to bend, to please, to survive. But true healing means knowing when not to bend. It means honoring your boundaries, sticking to your non-negotiables.

I've also learned to trust the intelligence of all three of my "brains" —my head, my heart, and my gut. The mind is logical. The heart is emotional. The gut is intuitive. When all three are aligned, that's when I feel most grounded, most whole.

I've come to understand the integration of logic and love, of mental clarity and emotional wisdom. And when the different parts of us converge, they become a true compass.

I've started listening to my gut the way I used to listen to a song, deeply, with reverence. I remember how my stomach would twist when my stepfather's anger filled the room. That was my body trying to protect me. That was wisdom. That was a checkpoint I didn't yet know how to trust. Now, I trust it.

That same trio—mind, heart, gut—shows up every time I perform. I've always felt nervous before stepping on stage, but that kind of nervousness is a friend. It says, *You care. You're alive. You're about to give something real.* My brain reminds me, *You've prepared.* My heart says, *Feel the music.* And my gut? It tells me when I've hit the note that truly matters.

I'm reminded of *The Wizard of Oz,* a story I never thought would speak to me as deeply as it does now. You need a brain to have courage. You need courage to have a heart. And when you bring them all together, you find your way home. Maybe that's a little corny for a brother from the hood, but it works for me.

These days, I believe mindfulness and body awareness should be taught in every school, right alongside math, science, and English. Trauma doesn't discriminate, and healing shouldn't either.

The Japanese have an art form called *Kintsugi*. It's the process of repairing broken pottery with gold. Every crack is honored, every fracture filled, not hidden, but highlighted. The piece becomes more beautiful, more valuable, because of what it's survived.

That's what I am.

That's what many of us are.

We are *Kintsugi people,* beautifully broken, but mended with intention and grace. That's the gift I've been given.

My story has given me the ability to walk into a room, see a young person, and feel what they need.

That gift has helped me create healing in all kinds of ways and carve a unique path from the rubble of my own pain. It helped me write music that reached the charts and healed people's hearts, including my own.

In 2024, I was awarded an honorary doctorate—not because I followed a traditional path, but because I turned pain into purpose. Even though pain and trauma threatened my mental and physical health, they did not get the final word.

Today, I am passionate about helping people MENifest their truth. That is not a typo. It's a word I coined that expresses what I hope men everywhere can discover if they carry pain from the past.

So what is *MENifesting*?

It's choosing love over fear.

It's trusting your own divine intelligence.

It's learning to hold yourself, even when no one else does.

It's becoming whole again, not *despite* your brokenness, but *because* of it.

This is my story.

This is my healing.

This is my offering.

ABOUT the AUTHOR

Dr. Vince Johnson is a speaker, educator, and inventor whose life's journey embodies the message of pain transformed into power and purpose. He has played and recorded with award winning musicians. Raised in Denver, Colorado, Vince found his voice – literally and metaphorically – through music, using it to rise above a childhood marked by trauma and adversity.

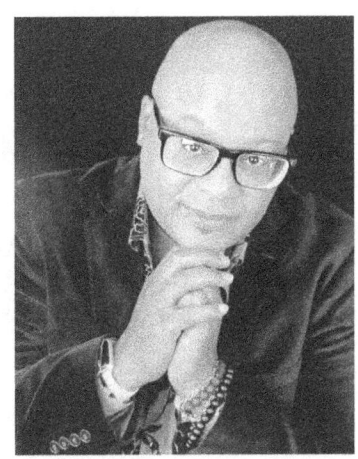

A patent holder in the field of healing technology, Vince blends science, spirituality, and sound to promote emotional wellness. He is the creator and host of a powerful podcast series focused on healing, growth, and transformation, and has worked with over 5,000 youth to inspire change through music and mentorship.

While Vince was signed to MTV Records, his song earned the #11 spot on Adult Contemporary Radio, and he has been employed by the world's first music software company, pioneering the way music and technology intersect for modern artists. A multi-instrumentalist and internationally touring performer, his work bridges generations, cultures, and consciousness.

In 2024, he was awarded an Honorary Ph.D. for his outstanding contribution to youth empowerment and trauma recovery. Today, Dr. Johnson's mission is simple but profound: help people MENifest their truth by choosing love over fear.

To learn more, visit: www.vincejohnsonjr.com

Chapter 14

Beauty Out of Ashes

Jonathan Dubrulle

A 24-year-old gay man just diagnosed with Schizaphrenia, gazing from the rooftop of Bellevue Hospital over the New York City skyline. Where is life going to take me? Am I going back to Belgium? Can I recover from this? Will I be like the caterpillar and become a beautiful butterfly, or all hope lost?

Growing Up in Louvain, Belgium

I grew up in a university town. My parents owned a driving school and did their best to succeed in life without degrees and to support their children financially.

I was a lovely kid who liked to walk around with a book in his mouth.

I was a genius at things in elementary school. When I was eight years old, I took an IQ test given by a psychologist in school, who said that I scored like a 14-year-old in the verbal part. But life was hard. My parents were not great at loving, but my grandma saved the day.

In my final year of elementary school, my teacher ran over to me in the gym and kissed me on the cheek, because I scored 100% on the final math exam. Both a kiss from a teacher and a perfect math exam score are unusual in Belgium.

My first love was Krishna, a Bernese mountain dog. I became a vegetarian at around 12 years old, which was unique, especially for guys. The gay theme emerged around age 13, and it was not met with love. High School was odd, but I could give a punch with words and I always had friends.

I started university at age 16, and I made university friends that I still have today, but I carried loneliness inside because I couldn't be fully myself and be appreciated.

Lost in Tokyo

In the final year of my Master's studies, I experimented with drugs, went out, and got selected for a reality TV show. The show was called *Lost in Tokyo*, and the story that I love most is how I got eliminated in the third episode.

We were supposed to grab a live eel out of an aquarium, kill it, and cut it open. I just couldn't. I said before the Japanese jury of 100 people, "I don't and won't kill animals. I won't." My refusal meant I couldn't win the €25,000 anymore.

A facet of my character, revealed at age 20: I love being brave and doing the right thing, even if it has repercussions.

Looking back, it was a marvelous experience, that included a free two-week trip to Tokyo, a night's stay in the Presidential suite of the Hilton, and the chance to learn how a TV show is made.

The Initial Cracks

At 19, I moved abroad for the first time, alone on an exchange semester in the city of Toulouse in the South of France. The experience was hard at times. While I was there,, I felt a little lump in my nipple and thought it might be a tumor. It was a cyst that could be sorted with meds.

That was the first time I realized that I experience things psychosomatically–feeling emotions physically in my body.. It happened again when I fell in love for the first time.

When my dog Hugo died, I was traveling in Cabo Verde and I suddenly got a high fever. A doctor came to the hotel and gave me an injection in my bum. The next day, she was surprised that my body temperature was fine again, which she said was unusual.

After graduating, I started a corporate career at Thomson Reuters, a Canadian multinational company.

When I started working full-time, I didn't yet know my physical limits. One weekend, I did a 10K run in 53 minutes. The next weekend, I did a 10-mile run that took place in a forest with very steep climbs and descents. About 200 meters before the finish, I stopped and walked. While walking to the car, people said that I looked pale. I started feeling unwell and felt tingling all over my body.

My dad drove me to the hospital, and I got the all clear. One week later, I went back to the gym and felt unwell again, so the gym staff called an ambulance. I stayed all night in the emergency room, and doctors found a conduction error in my heart. I was advised to never run another marathon, but I could still exercise.

A couple of weeks later, I left to start a business graduate program in London. I remember feeling so stressed that I found myself lying on the bathroom floor in the Canary Wharf building, listening to calming meditation music.

From London, I moved to Geneva. Because of ongoing stress, my heart would skip beats. Even in the bathtub, I would feel as if my heart rate was half of a normal heartbeat.

The Healing Journey in Singapore

Next stop was Singapore; I was far away from home and had the freedom and space to explore who I really was in my heart. Singapore, a country that I had never visited before, was 7000 miles away from home. I was 22, but looked way younger, with a mind that could handle the world but with a body that hadn't yet lived much life.

On January 22, my 23rd birthday, I was riding in a taxi and asking the universe what my gift would be when I opened an expat magazine that was in the pouch in front of me. My eyes were glued to an ad on one of the pages about a chiropractic healing practice called Innate.

I started going to sessions three times a week. In March, Simon, a recent graduate who was 28 years old, started working on me. I fell in love with him easily. When everything aligned, from romantic to sexual to spiritual connection, I knew for sure that I was gay.

However, nothing illegal happened. It was unrequited love, a mandatory experience for a lot of people, but it hurt badly. I felt pain in my body for months and couldn't sleep more than four to five hours a night.

I finally said to him, in the hallway of the practice in Camden Medical Center, "I think I am in love with you."

To which he replied, "Just like friends?"

I said, "No, not just like friends," and that was the end of the conversation. I found it odd that he continued working on me after I told him I was in love with him.

I kept going until my deceased grandmother appeared to me in my dream and said, "Laat los," which means "let go" in Dutch. I wrote a goodbye letter to Simon and handed it over to him during our last session. The last sentence of that letter said, "You'll always be my first love."

I flew home for my summer holiday to Belgium and told my family and friends that I had fallen in love and realized that I was gay. My dad was shocked, and still today, he struggles with it. In January 2025, he said, "I can accept two women holding hands, but not two men."

His philosophy that was shared in Singapore, where sex between two men was illegal until 2022, but not sex with two women.

In June 2025, my dad continued to spread the gay hatred.

You're not a bloke because you're a homo, but you couldn't tell because you're not effeminate.

Months later, Simon showed up twice at the new practice I was going to in Network, Spinal Chiropractic. The second time I saw him, he said that he was there to give me closure and that he wasn't gay.

Looking back, I am not impressed by myself for making the

connection that I was gay at 23. But, since my dad was a Mormon and considering the spirit of the time 15 years ago, it is understandable.

I felt I couldn't flourish in such a conservative environment, so I moved to New York City and started a new role in Corporate Strategy.

The Total Collapse in New York City

In January 2011, when I moved from the equator to New York City, at the opposite end of the world, I traded tropical weather for freezing weather. The tone was set for an ice-cold experience.

Walking to work in the snow from 350 W. 43rd Street to the Times Square office, I would feel the cold on my skin and think about Simon. Little did I know that the experience of unrequited love, my genes, my identity issues, and an unhelpful Harvard Business School SVP would push me to a breaking point.

Three weeks before I reached that point, the psychosis had begun on a flight from NYC to Denver. While traveling to Denver to attend a Transformational Gate healing event hosted by Dr. Donny Epstein, I started hearing voices.

I was convinced that I had a chip in my brain. The plane connected through Chicago, and I was convinced that I would be on the Oprah show as an interesting case. While the plane ascended through the clouds, I heard a whisper saying, "Trust in the love of God."

On the evening of March 6th, back in New York City, I had such a headache that I couldn't sleep. My head felt like it was torturing me. After a sleepless night, the voice said that it would kill me if I didn't go to the office. I decided to go.

In the office, I called Emily, the SVP who I'd felt was teasing me about my sexuality. I said, "I will get you for this."

She called me a child. I pulled the fire alarm, which I thought would end the show in my unsettled state of mind, then I went up to the executive floor.

The receptionist recognized me and buzzed me in. I went to Carol, a VP, and started hysterically crying. "I can't do this anymore," I told her.

I was taken into a meeting room, where the Global Head of HR and another colleague sat next to me.

I warned them, "Don't come closer because I don't know what I will do."

They got the message. Next, the security officer of the building came, put plastic zip tie handcuffs around my wrist, and led me to the service elevator. When I stepped out of the elvator, an ambulance was waiting, and the Director of Graduate Programs, Elizabth, was waiting in the ambulance. I sat down and said, "She is just in it for the fame." That was the craziest line I think I've ever said in my entire life.

I would stay in Bellevue Hospital for 17 days. A challenging environment, but I was safe. The oddest experience was a roommate who wrote a love letter in his own blood. He was moved to a different room.

My mom flew in immediately from Europe. The CEO's driver was waiting for her at the airport and drove her to the hotel that had been booked for her. The handling of the situation by Thomson Reuters was exceptional.

Nevertheless, the experience was harsh for a 24-year-old who looked like a 20-year-old.

On the plane back to Brussels, where I had decided to move after I was released, I couldn't sit still, to the embarrassment of my sister, who had flown in as well. The co-pilot came to check on me, and paramedics came onto the plane when we arrived on Belgian soil. They asked if I took meds, and I said, "Risperidone," which was given to me in the hospital.

They responded, "Oh, psychiatric patient." People were waking up and looking over, but I made it off the plane without any further incidents. That would become the start of a transition.

I would continue to be hospitalized for a couple of weeks in Belgium. During that time, my friends would visit me in the hospital. After I was released, others would meet me for lunch. A support system is such a blessing when the times get dark, and they reminded me that there is always hope on the horizon.

Maturing Safely on the Sofa

During the next 13 years, I would safely mature, mainly on the sofa in my mom's home. After New York, I would still work seven months for Thomson Reuters in Brussels, but I decided to quit, despite the financial consequences and loss of insurance provided by the company.

I completed a bachelor's degree in health sciences at The Open Universit I learned Spanish, and began to volunteer again, and do some traveling, which I always loved. The pace of life would slow down so I could process, and get used to living life with schizophrenia.

I would gain weight and even became obese at one point. My stretch marks still testify to that. The first years were the hardest, marked by a constant frown above my eyes, but *paso a paso–one step at a time*–things started to improve very slowly.

In time, I invested in a student studio and rented it out. It was hard work, but I bought it in 2014 and sold it in 2024, which turned out to be a great financial decision that had a real impact on my financial well-being.

Moving to Madrid

In September 2024, I moved to Madrid to attend chiropractic school. Two days before my departure, Pope Saint Francis came to visit my hometown for the 600th anniversary of the University where I studied. It felt like a blessing to see him on his final trip before he left this world.

I was passionate about the chiropractic technique that had impacted my life, Network Spinal. I fell in love for a second time, with someone named Emilio, but the stress made my head too busy again with voices. I had to leave school, which made me cry because things were ruined again.

In Madrid, I dated guys. One I met at church. I had a crush on him, but he just lied in the end and hurt me badly. Another was very attractive, but sexy love is not love.

While living in Madrid, things started to change at a rapid pace. I could cry again, feel chills, enjoy being myself, find my sense of style, lose weight, and get fit. I followed an alternative path and got certified in the Spinal Flow technique in January 2025.

The gift is often different than what I expected. I came here for chiropractic school, but the gift was falling in love with Madrid and deciding to stay here.

I set up a chiropractic practice in my apartment and started to become the embodiment of the person that I wanted to be. I started to travel and attract luck. Over Christmas, while traveling back to my hometown, my Tom Ford sunglasses would be fixed, polished, and fitted for free. I travelled to London, Paris, and Leiria, and received three free hotel upgrades in a row.

When I was flying back from Berlin to Madrid, I was even allowed to travel back to Madrid without the passport that I had lost at the airport. When you have positive vibes, with a pleasant demeanor, with the right words, the world responds differently.

My dad came to visit at the end of May, when I bought my own apartment in Madrid. His gay hatred and negative intentions were unwelcome. In Barajas Airport, when I said goodbye to him, he said that he was worried I would fall in love with someone who was just interested in my money. He added that he needed more time. I told him that 15 years is long enough.

I think he will be happier not having to face his gay son anymore. I gave him two fashion magazines with me on the cover, hoping that he would see that I'm a beautiful man inside and out.

Magazine Writing & Fashion Photography

My mental health has improved. With a schizophrenia diagnosis, past heart issues, and asthma, it is essential for me to counteract the health impact of meds. I quit smoking seven years ago, I eat way more healthily by cooking daily and eating more veggies, carrying a water bottle to stay hydrated. I work out twice a week at the gym and I'm focusing on living my best life. I don't drink alcohol–not even the free ones you get in restaurants–and don't do drugs.

I started writing articles for Brainz Magazine, Passion Vista, and Health & Wellbeing Magazine. I have a cute healing practice in Madrid. I love traveling in business class with Iberia airlines around Europe, attending retreats, and doing photo shoots.

I am back at my ideal weight now. In May 2025, I did a seaside photo shoot in St Leonards in the United Kingdom. It was a brilliant day, the sun was shining, and a seal showed up in the water. Now I have pictures to look back on when I'm 50 or 70 years old.

I submitted pictures to some fashion magazines and was requested for the cover of several, including *Enzomnia Magazine* from Barcelona featuring the theme, "Beauty with Schizophrenia". I have also been featured on the cover of fashion magazines from Amsterdam, Barcelona, Japan, Kyiv, LA, London, Milan, New York City, and Paris. But there are always things to manage. I am extremely sensitive to heat and stress. Sometimes when I feel unwell, I need to take a taxi home. That is a practical advantage in big cities like Singapore, New York City, and Madrid; you just raise your hand and go back home. And I don't need to travel by ambulance anymore.

A Trip to Auschwitz and Ukraine in June 2025

In late June of 2025, I visited the birthplace of my paternal grandmother, Krakow, Poland. It was my first visit, and I was surprised by the beautiful charm of the old town.

After having a vegetarian dinner in the Bhajan Café, the waitress said there was a temple in the basement and that I could visit with my shoes off. In the Hindu temple, I reached out to divinity as I was going to Ukraine the next day, a country still at war.

Walking back, I remembered a church that stuck in my mind. I went in, looked at the light-coloured ceiling, and prayed that all would go well during my travels, hoping that the video and fashion shoot would be safe and have a real-world impact.

But first, I visited the darkest reminder on planet Earth of how evil humans can get. On a guided tour from Krakow to Auschwitz, I heard nauseating stories about how 1.5 million people were gassed in five years' time.

I took the leap of faith to go and visit Ukraine, a country at war with Russia for over three years. Some people didn't understand, as I was risking my life. But being brave and wanting to make a difference includes calculated risk-taking.

I took wartime insurance, Ukrainian health insurance, installed the AirAlarmUkraine app, and booked a hotel. Then I took a bus from Krakow to Lviv in Ukraine.

Lviv is the biggest city in the west of Ukraine, and given the longer distance to Russia, it was the safest bet for a first-time visitor.

The seven-hour bus trip included several hours spent at the Polish-Ukrainian border. It's an annoying part of the trip. I arrived at night, and given the curfew, the only option was to take a taxi directly to the hotel.

The next day, I met at St. George Cathedral with my photographer and videographer, Andrey. He came by car, as he said it was too dangerous on foot, since police ask for the papers of men and force them to fight on the front line if they are over 25 years old.

The best was saved for last. Andrey and I went to a newly created graveyard for the military personnel who died during the conflict that started on February 22, 2022. I was allowed to place a candle for a soldier whose DNA could not be identified.

No one was allowed to say how many people were buried there, but there were thousands of graves and flags waving in the wind. The images in my mind are unforgettable and touched my heart.

While we were walking back, buses of military personnel and families were arriving, along with a brass ensemble, to pay their last respects for a new hero who had fallen.

My Perspective & Advice

I learned about doing the right thing even if it is hard. When maturing, my focus shifted from myself to other people. I love reaching out to friends and family, giving affordable Spinal Flow Technique sessions for the Madrilenian community, and influencing and inspiring the world through my writing and social media posts on Instagram, Threads, Facebook, and LinkedIn. Even walking through airport security, a glove fell off a baby onto the floor. The veiled mother didn't notice, so I picked it up and gave it to her. Even that small act felt significant.

I am a healer in my soul and love writing, traveling the world, being on the radio, and posting on social media. The butterfly ring I always wear is a reminder of transformation; from the caterpillar to the butterfly. Its natural beauty and strength resonate with my core.

My Advice to Others:

1. Discover who you are romantically, sexually, and spiritually. Knowing yourself sets you up to impact the world.
2. People should be free to live and be themselves. Accept people for who they are.
3. People in the dark have a lack of clarity and understanding, and darkness has to be stopped.

At some point in life, you transcend your diagnoses and love who you are, and focus on your soul mission. In my case, to battle darkness with a guided approach and blessed by the hand of God.

In memoriam of Vinzie the cat (May 2025).

ABOUT the AUTHOR

A Leader Who Believes that life should be about enjoying yourself, after finding out who you are and loving yourself.

As a Model, Magazine Writer, and Former Healer, he loves contributing to the world, especially in teaching people better behavior.

Times are changing, and he's publishing, *Join the Veggie Snake Club Book* soon.

Social Link:
linktr.ee/jdubrulle

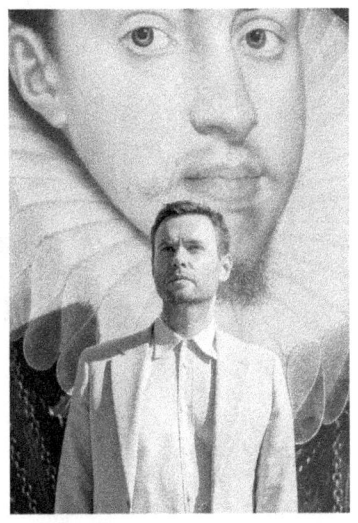

Chapter 15

For The Love Of Men
Natalie Goodfellow

"*Oh, you are so sensitive!!!*" These words have echoed in my soul for as long as I can remember. Being a sensitive child in my world during the '70s and '80s was a challenge. The perception that I was weak for *feeling* and even weaker for *expressing* these feelings has followed me throughout my life. I knew how difficult it was to be a female with strong emotions. However, I never truly appreciated what it was to be a male with strong emotions until I became a mother of two boys.

The two people who always showed the most acceptance for my sensitivity were the two men I loved first in my life: my father and my brother. They were always compassionate and held space for me during my times of emotional highs and lows. I did not feel weak in their presence. I felt seen and accepted, although I believe at a deeper level, they too viewed my sensitivity as weakness.

Feelings are as natural as breathing, yet so dreaded, so feared by so many, especially men. *Men don't cry,* is equivalent to *women don't experience pain in childbirth.* If men don't cry, then that implies they don't feel. But they do feel, and they have had to repress their feelings for years. I heard many years ago that there are enough toxins in tears to kill a small rodent. If this is a fact, just imagine what repression is doing to the physiological and neurological systems of our men.

It is our ability to think and feel that differentiates us from our relatives in the animal kingdom. Yes, humans have a primal survival response to *react* as animals do, but we also have the capacity to *respond* via our ability to think and feel. Yet this is a skill that, although completely natural, is a mystery to many of us. Emotions are at the forefront of who we are. Instead of fearing them, we need to develop a relationship with them, accept them, understand their purpose in our lives, and give them permission to be felt.

I am entering the *crone* phase of my life. This is the phase of life where one feels the desire to give back to society the cumulative wisdom of one's experiences. A time to speak out and act in hopes of making a difference in the lives of others.

Mental health issues affect all of us, not just individually but collectively. It is essential that we take the time to understand the underlying issues and root causes of this important area of our health, as a one-size-fits-all approach does not resolve the issues facing women, children, or men.

I have dedicated 30 years of my life to teaching elementary students in Canada. During my last three years, most of the challenges in the classroom came from the males in my classes. I retired in 2019, just before COVID-19, but the escalation of behavioral concerns after COVID in the primary grades, kindergarten and first grade continues to be heartbreaking and astonishing.

What is happening to our little boys? If this is happening to them at their tender age, what will be in store for them in adolescence or adulthood?

Our educational system is doing a huge disservice to our male students by not addressing the unique needs of boys. Physiological differences between males and females go beyond genitalia. It is common knowledge among parents, caregivers, and teachers that life for many boys is all about action and adventure. They are programmed to move, and many are fascinated with anything that moves.

> "Scientists used to think this stereotypical boy behavior was the result of socialization, but we now know that the greater motivation for movement is biologically wired in the male brain."
>
> — Louann Brizendine, *The Male Brain*, 2010, p.22

How many times have parents said, "He is sweet and cuddly one minute and the next minute he's squirming out of my arms!"?

Then comes the fear from the parent that their child is hyperactive or has ADHD. The reason for the higher activity in males is due to their developing hormone levels, which occur between birth and age ten as much as it does when a male reaches puberty. Brizendine's book has opened my eyes to how differently men's minds and bodies operate. (She has also written *The Female Brain*.) The information in this book is fascinating and a valuable resource for educators, parents, and women in relationships with men.

Schools are expecting males to succeed in a system that claims to "meet the needs of all" without even understanding those needs. We send children to school as young as three-and-a-half years old in Ontario, Canada, with the hope of introducing them earlier to the educational system and providing them with the opportunity to learn sooner. But I remember as a kindergarten teacher how we dreaded the junior kindergarten students during September. We often referred to these students as a group of squirrels. Their ability to follow instructions, sit, and listen was very limited. Looking back, I now see how we did not consider the fact that these children, especially boys, are not developmentally ready to sit and follow directions for long periods. Today, we think even less of the importance of providing them with daily physical education. Many schools don't let their students go outside during recess in the winter due to icy yard conditions and the fear of students getting hurt. Kids spend much of their school day in low physical activity situations when they need to expend energy running, moving, and developing their muscles.

The impact of these decisions is far-reaching. We are essentially diagnosing, labelling, and medicating students (primarily males) because they are unable to sit, follow instructions, and comply with our commands. Their need to move should not be viewed as undesired behavior; it is a physical need. When we repress this need, we also repress the production and release of other hormones and chemicals essential to their emotional development.

We inadvertently create a dislike for school in these young males as young as six years of age. Boys are hands-on, boys are active, and boys learn differently than girls. What we are doing is repressing their growth, shaming them for who they are, and medicating them to comply with a "sit and listen" philosophy of learning.

Our sedentary lifestyle has impacted everyone's health in numerous ways. However, this is especially evident in males and their mental health. As stated earlier, movement encourages the natural flow of hormones and blood flow, producing *feel-good* chemicals in our brains, and encouraging the production and release of male hormones. Boys who don't have a healthy means of dispensing their physical energy often get labelled as having behavior problems when they merely have a buildup of physical energy they need to exert.

When they go home, unless they are in organized sports, most don't engage in any physical activity either. They are living a sedentary life, one that is being imposed by the social restructuring of society. Kids don't go outside and play anymore due to the fear of stranger danger and the influx of computer games. The skyrocketing cost of organized sports is also making this option a limited one for families. The results of ignoring the core physiological needs of males impact their mental health at an early age.

It is time for the school system to place value on emotional intelligence rather than only academic intelligence. Teaching children the vocabulary associated with the most natural part of being a human, emotions, can help to normalize their experiences. Providing them with the skills and strategies to deal with emotional experiences would be lifesaving. It's time to make emotional education as common and available in schools as sex education is.

The following is not a derogatory statement towards men. It is a fact based on my personal experience: Much of the pain in my life has been connected to men. Men whom I have loved dearly, and who have loved me reciprocally. Good men, hardworking, caring, and supportive in the ways they knew how to be. But most of all, loving men. Yet the common denominator that led to the pain in my life and the lives of others in my family was the pain in the hearts of the men we loved. These incredible men became overwhelmed with the uncertainties of life and the discomfort of experiencing "Raw Emotions" without having the ability, the skills, or the awareness to handle and process them. These raw, human emotions and the inability of the men in my family to process them, led to addictive and avoidant behavior, which has caused enormous heartbreak.

On November 17, 2001, my world changed forever, not just my world, the world of three generations of my family. My brother had just become a father to a beautiful, healthy baby girl in September. Then suddenly, one Saturday morning in November, he collapsed on the job site where he was working alongside my father. Just like that, he was gone, dead.

Everything changed. Everything! How could this have happened? What exactly happened?

As it turns out, my brother had been told at age 28 that he needed heart surgery. The day he died, he was less than one month away from his 33rd birthday, and no one knew about this medical recommendation. He was born with a heart defect, and my parents took him to the doctor annually until he was old enough to go on his own. But the last time he went to the doctor, he heard information that his emotions did not know how to handle, and his way of dealing with the news was to avoid it.

That day in November, when I received the call about his death, I literally lost my mind. I was running around my house screaming and roaring and collapsing to the ground. Then I looked up at my two boys, who were three and six at the time, and said to myself, "Natalie, you must get yourself together." I wasn't just reacting to the death of my brother. As upset as I was, I knew I would be ok. I was no stranger to death. I had experienced the death of my beautiful baby girl eight years prior to my brother's death, and I knew I would come through. But what about my parents, particularly my father? My father had just been through a decade of loss. The loss of his mother, brother-in-law, friend, business, and now the loss of his son. Just as I expected, he kept his grief to himself and numbed his pain with alcohol. The men who had always allowed me to express emotion wouldn't let themselves do the same.

After spending time reflecting on these experiences and working on my own healing, I realized these behaviors were unintentional. Unintentional in the sense that they were not meant to cause pain to other family members. Also, unintentional was the way they were passed down by previous generations. Behaviors that have been ingrained in many men, not just the men in my family, who use avoidance as a means of handling emotions.

I have since learned many things about men. Men's strength can be a mask for pain. Many connect vulnerability with shame. I also understand that anger in a man can be sadness in disguise. The one thing I know for sure is that most men love deeper than they let on.

Societal beliefs continue to shift related to men and emotions. This is a good thing. Men, like women, feel things. They feel as deeply as women do. However, women tend to reach out for support, and they can generally ask others for help. It has been my experience that men do not have this same connection within themselves or their networks. Many men do not allow themselves to feel vulnerable, and as a result of this emotional isolation, they often experience profound loneliness.

Teaching people how to regulate their emotions is crime prevention, it's addiction prevention, as well as a means of reducing the number of fatherless families in our society. Not addressing men's needs means children will grow up and continue the cycle all over again. This cyclical devastation can be changed through awareness and education. However, a crucial question worth asking would be, *Is this awareness and education viewed as a priority in our culture?*

Three things are certain in life: death, taxes, and change. Change is often perceived as negative. However, much growth and positivity can come from change. We can decide to view change as negative or as a means of evolving. I believe it is time for greater change to occur in our society, and the change I am referring to involves the rearing, socializing, educating, and loving of our males.

It's time to change the conversation about men's mental health. Societal beliefs take time to shift, but it's time to take steps towards this shift. We can ask ourselves: How are we parenting our boys? Do we parent our sons differently from our daughters? Why are fathers more likely to be harder on their sons than their daughters? Is there the perception that they need to "toughen" their boys up to survive in this world?

How are we teaching boys? What expectations do we have for males compared to females in school? In sports? What about the dating world? Many women are no longer looking for providers. They are looking for partners. Yet there is still a demographic of men who are raised and conditioned only to be providers and protectors.

Change requires a group effort and time, but it must start somewhere. Parents, spouses and partners, school systems, government policies, and the workplace can each play an important role. However, the best place to exhibit a change like this is during childhood. Effective change in parenting, education, and the relationships between men and women can be essential starting points to encourage healthier support systems for generations of men.

It is crucial that parents realize the importance of understanding the needs of their children. However, to meet our children's needs, we must become aware of our own unmet needs and triggers. Supporting the whole child provides emotional security and healthy development, providing a foundation that gives children the ability to develop resilience and perseverance.

The current research on neuroplasticity suggests that we can reprogram, essentially rewire our brains at all stages of life. Knowing the importance of early intervention though, do we as parents understand the importance of our role? Are we in touch with our own emotions? Do we have the tools and support to navigate challenges in our own lives? These are skills that must be taught. They are essential in the development of a healthy society and in creating happy lives and a functioning economy. Most people take more time to plan and prepare for a vacation than they spend preparing to become parents.

The U.S. Surgeon General's advisory document from August 2024 identifies how parental stress has essentially become an epidemic, impacting the mental health of children. Thirty years ago, when I became a working mom, I experienced this stress while trying to juggle work and parenting. I was fortunate enough to work part-time until my boys were in school full-time. Today's economy does not support the needs of many families. Part-time work is not an option for many; in fact, multiple jobs are often required to make ends meet. Parents, in many cases, are only able to provide the basic necessities of life for their children.

We are a society whose nervous systems are living in survival mode. The hustle culture no longer applies to the workplace; it is how many families function daily. This constant being "on" and needing to do, and perform, is activating the nervous systems of both parents and kids. There is no time to rest and digest. No time to experience and process emotions. We are depriving our families of the most basic emotional need, the need to connect. Yet, as a society, do we support parents and caregivers? Do we value the raising of children?

"Raising children is sacred work. It should matter to all of us," the U.S. Surgeon General stated. When parents are impacted, children are impacted. This impact has dire social repercussions on the future of society. It is time to allocate resources to educate, support, and prevent mental health crises rather than treating them. It is my opinion that this is the responsibility of employers as well as the government.

We have gone from an authoritative approach to a passive means of raising children. Neither is what children need. They need leaders, and unfortunately, the males in so many families have been left without male leaders. What do good leaders do? Good leaders inspire, communicate effectively, build strong relationships, and foster a positive and inclusive environment, while making sound decisions and taking responsibility for their actions. Good leaders are positive, encouraging, and uplifting. They praise employees for a job well done, taking time to coach and train if there are lapses in performance. In good times and bad, good leaders bring out the best in their employees by encouraging them to be their very best.

Adam Grant states in his blog, Qualtrics, "Good leaders build products. Great leaders build cultures. Good leaders deliver results. Great leaders develop people. Good leaders have vision. Great leaders have values. Good leaders are role models at work. Great leaders are role models in life." (Grant, 2022)

This kind of leadership at home, as well as in schools and government, is what children need. However, in many cases, this is not what our children are receiving. Children benefit from and need mothers and fathers in their lives. If this is not possible, they need male and female role models with whom they can connect. When stress leads to relationship failure, separation leads to more disturbances for children. Once again, learning how to navigate this stress with a support system is good for families, employers, and society.

We have come a long way in society with women claiming their independence and space in the workplace, politics, and family. My grandmothers and my mother were women who were reliant on their husbands for their survival. I was not, as I had other options available to me.

I divorced after 24 years of marriage, and I landed on my feet because I had an education and the ability to provide for myself and my child. I am not alone in this reality. This is the reality for many women today. Many women can leave marriages that are no longer in their best interest, and they have the right to do so. Sometimes I question if we do so too easily. We live in a cancel culture, where it is easy to dismiss what doesn't align with us. However, there are consequences to this dismissal that cannot be overlooked.

The role of men today is not so much that of protector and provider. Women, in most cases, are looking for partners. Emotional, intellectual, social, parental, and family partners with whom to share the responsibilities of life.

There seems to be a huge divide between men and women and our roles in society. I have had the opportunity to speak with coaches working with men. Jason Tremblay from JayT Consulting in Quebec, Canada, confirms that "Stress and anxiety are increasingly prevalent in the dad community and many men don't feel the women in their lives are fully supporting them, as there is still a misconception that men are unbreakable." Is it possible that women, in their desire to be seen as equal to men, believed they needed to become more masculine? Is there possibly an imbalance of masculine and feminine energy occurring in relationships today?

I often hear and have said it myself, "Men don't communicate." Instead of cancelling them, why not take the opportunity to teach them, model it for them, and understand that this is something they may not have had the chance to learn. A woman's role as partner, mother, sister, daughter, and friend can be powerful in providing emotional space for the men in her life.

Today, I am proud to say that I am still the sensitive being that I was all those years ago. Today, however, I am completely comfortable with my sensitivity. I have developed the awareness and emotional intelligence necessary to navigate strong emotions.

I can't help but wonder how differently life would have turned out if my brother had shared his uncomfortable thoughts about the surgery he needed with those of us who loved him. I also think about how different the last 17 years of my father's life, after my brother's death, could have been if he had known how to express his grief.

Emotions, sensitivity, compassion, and empathy are not bad words. They are what make us human, and they are the ties that bind us together in our relationships. They are words that our world needs to become familiar with in order to move forward as a progressive, responsible, and evolved society.

ABOUT the AUTHOR

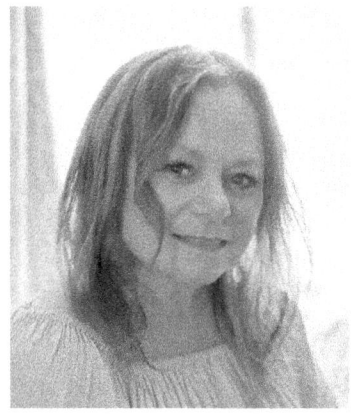

Natalie Goodfellow lives in Martintown, Ontario, Canada. Natalie has spent the past 35 years as a teacher, mother, stepmother, foster mother, and grandmother. She has recently written a children's book on developing spiritual awareness called *Grammy Who Is Guss?* Natalie currently works as an Awareness Coach and is passionate about empowering children, teens, and adults to use awareness and mindset shifts to live fulfilling lives. Natalie is also a certified Parent Coach and Life Coach and the founder of Triple R Coaching. Her coaching modality focuses on three steps to help individuals shift from surviving to thriving: recognize, replace, and repair. You can find her at nataliegoodfellow.com or on Instagram and Facebook at @TripleR_Coaching.

Visit our Website

Visit our facebook

Visit our Instagram

Acknowledgements

With deep gratitude, we acknowledge Dr. Katherine Humphreys for her invaluable support of the authors throughout the writing process, offering guidance and encouragement every step of the way.

Our heartfelt thanks also go to the Red Thread team, whose dedication and vision made this project possible. The support of Sierra Melcher has been vital at every step of the process.

To all the authors, we honor your courage, vulnerability, and commitment in bringing men's mental health into the light; your voices are the heartbeat of this book.

We are also grateful to our early readers: Mimi Rich, Michael Pund, David Letiecq, Paul L. Symmonds, Dr. Will Folberth and Brendee Melcher, for your thoughtful insights and reflections that strengthened these pages.

Finally, special thanks to Emily Sutherland, our editor, for her care, clarity, and steady hand in shaping this book into its fullest form.

Review this Book

Enjoyed MENtal Health? Your feedback means the world! If the book resonated with you, inspired you, or offered some-thing meaningful, we'd truly appreciate it if you left a review on Amazon or GoodReads. Your feedback helps others discover the book—and it directly supports the author's work.

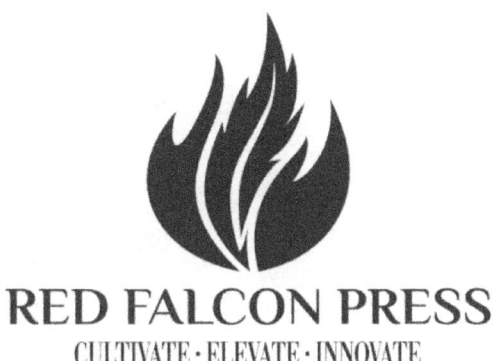

RED FALCON PRESS
CULTIVATE · ELEVATE · INNOVATE

About the Publisher

Red Thread Publishing is an award-winning indie press dedicated to amplifying powerful, authentic nonfiction voices. In our first five years, we've published more than 65 books, supported over 320 authors from 30 countries, and celebrated 38 book awards, proof of the impact and quality behind every title we produce.

We publish through two imprints: **Red Falcon Press**, which welcomes all genders and champions silenced and marginalized voices, and **Red Thread Books**, founded with the mission of helping 10,000 women become successful authorpreneurs and thought leaders.

Our passionate team is committed to guiding authors through every step of the journey so their stories not only get published but make a lasting impact. To explore our growing library or learn how to work with us, visit **www.redthreadbooks.com**

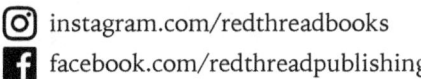

instagram.com/redthreadbooks
facebook.com/redthreadpublishing

Other books
Red Thread Collaborative Anthologies

∼

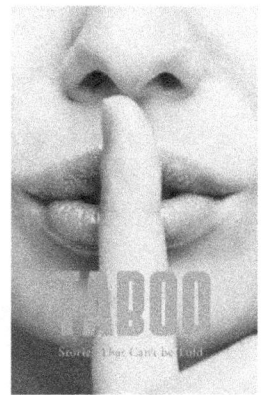

Taboo: Stories That Can't Be Told

∼

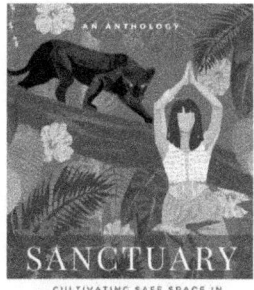

Sactuary: Cultivating Safe Space in Sisterhood; Rediscovering the Power that Unites Us

∼

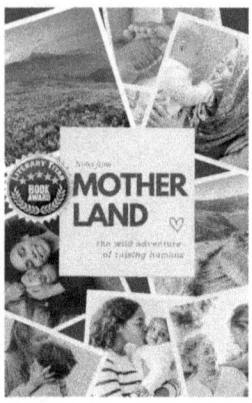

Notes From Motherland: The Wild Adventure of Raising Humans

∼

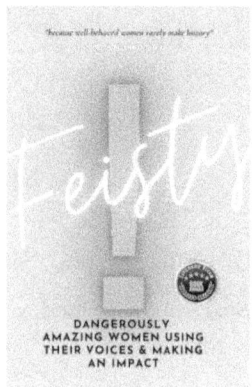

FEISTY: Dangerously Amazing Women Using Their Voices & Making An Impact

∼

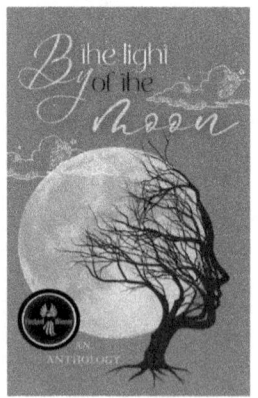

By the Light of the Moon

www.ingramcontent.com/pod-product-compliance
Lightning Source LLC
Chambersburg PA
CBHW020541030426
42337CB00013B/932